Bone Marrow and Blood Stem Cell TRANSPLANTS

A Guide for Patients and Their Loved Ones

Other books written by Susan K. Stewart

The Spanish version of this book, *Trasplantes de Médula Ósea y de Células Progenitoras en Sangre Periférica: Una Guía Para Pacientes*

*Autologous Stem Cell Transplants:
A Handbook for Patients*

(in English and Spanish)

*Graft-versus-Host Disease:
What to Know, What to Do*

(in English and Spanish)

*CAR T-CELL THERAPY:
What Expect Before, During and After*

You can order these books online at bmtinfonet.org/books
or by phoning 888-597-7674
Outside US phone 847-433-3313

Bone Marrow and Blood Stem Cell TRANSPLANTS

A Guide for Patients and Their Loved Ones

By Susan K. Stewart

Illustrated by Norm Bendell

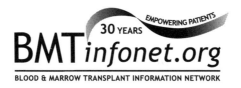

1548 Old Skokie Rd, Highland Park, IL 60035
phone: 847-433-3313   toll-free: 888-597-7674
email: help@bmtinfonet.org
Website: bmtinfonet.org

Copyright © 2002 Revised 2006, 2012, 2015, 2017, 2020

Funding provided by Gamida-Cell and by an unrestricted educational grant from Pharmacyclics, an AbbVie Company and Janssen Biotech, Inc.

Acknowledgements

Writing this book was not a solo effort. The generosity of many wonderful people helped make this book a reality.

I would especially like to thank:

Patrick J. Stiff MD who donated countless hours providing me with background material, reviewing drafts of the book, tirelessly responding to my many questions, and clarifying many technical details.

Martin S. Tallman MD, a warm, caring doctor and a personal friend who supported me first through my transplant, and afterwards as a medical advisor on this book.

Our wonderful scientific advisors for this edition:
Stephanie Lee MD, MPH, Fred Hutchinson Cancer Research Center
Navneet Majhail MD, MS, Cleveland Clinic
Steven Pavletic MD, National Cancer Institutes
Marcie Riches MD, MS, UNC Lineberger Comprehensive Cancer Center
Karen Syrjala PhD, Fred Hutchinson Cancer Research Center
Julie Vose MD, MBA, University of Nebraska Medical Center

Norm Bendell, whose illustrations appear throughout the book. Thanks, Norm, for helping to lighten up a very difficult text.

Kim Kultgen, who worked tirelessly on the design of this book to make it a pleasure to read.

The transplant recipients and caregivers quoted throughout the book who generously shared their experience and insights.

The wonderful staff at BMT InfoNet who reviewed and edited countless drafts.

And finally, to my husband and son whose patience and support helped make this book possible.

Thank you all!

This book is dedicated
to

Ruth Krueger

My mother, mentor and constant source of support.

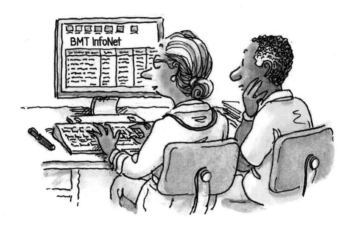

Visit BMTinfonet.org

Our website is your gateway to detailed information about what to expect before, during and after your transplant. Popular features include:

- **Transplant Basics:** how to prepare for transplant and how to manage issues that can arise during and after treatment

- **Emotional support** for transplant recipients and caregivers

- **Facts about nearly 200 transplant centers** including staff, number of transplants performed, accreditation and diseases treated

- **Video Learning Library** with extensive information about transplantation

- **Resource Directory** with links to financial help, disease information and more

You can also phone us toll-free at 888-597-7674.

We're with you every step of the way!

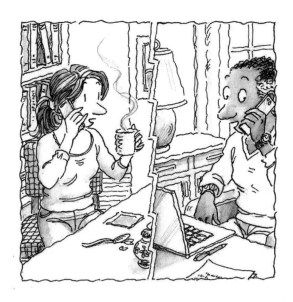

Caring Connections
Peer Support Program

If you or a loved one is going to have a transplant, chances are you are feeling scared and overwhelmed.

BMT InfoNet's **Caring Connections Program** can help.

More than 1,000 transplant recipients and their family members have volunteered to provide support for others facing a transplant.

Talk with people who:

- have been through a transplant
- understand how you feel
- can provide non-medical information and emotional support
- can offer tips for coping with the needs of family members, household and job responsibilities and more.

In most cases, our Caring Connections Program can connect you with someone who had the same diagnosis, same type of transplant and is approximately the same age.

If you are a family member of a patient, you can use the Caring Connections Program too!

Request a Caring Connection online at bmtinfonet.org/caring-connection or phone 888-597-7674.

Someone in our community of volunteers is looking forward to talking with you!

Table of Contents

1. History of Transplantation — 1
2. An Introduction to Transplantation — 7
3. Choosing a Transplant Center — 19
4. Finding a Donor — 31
5. Being a Donor — 35
6. Insurance and Fundraising — 45
7. Emotional Challenges — 51
8. When Your Child Needs a Transplant — 65
9. Preparative/Conditioning Regimen — 85
10. Graft-versus-Host Disease — 95
11. Infection — 111
12. Nutrition — 123
13. Relieving Pain — 137
14. Family Caregiver — 151
15. Planning for Survivorship — 167
16. Late Effects in Adults and Children — 177
17. Sexual Health after Transplant — 195
18. Family Planning — 201

Appendices
    A. About Blood Cells   205
    B. Understanding Blood Tests   209

Glossary of Terms   213

Index   219

More BMT InfoNet Literature   241

Dear Friend,

In 1988, after being diagnosed with leukemia, my doctor recommended a bone marrow transplant. I'd never heard of a bone marrow transplant and hadn't a clue as to what bone marrow or stem cells were and why they are important.

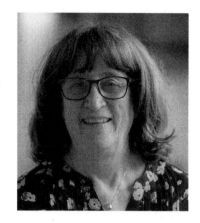

I was confused and overwhelmed. All the medical terms used to describe the treatment were new to me. Often, I was so lost I couldn't even figure out the right questions to ask! After recovering from my transplant, I met other survivors and learned my experience was not unique.

This book is written by and for patients with the help of many doctors, nurses, social workers, transplant recipients and their families. It's designed to translate into plain English the medical information you'll receive before, during and after your transplant.

There's no getting around it. Blood stem cell transplantation is a big, confusing subject. There is a lot of information to absorb in this book. Take it at your own pace.

Throughout the book you will find quotations from transplant recipients and their family caregivers — real people who faced the same challenges that now lie before you. They will tell you firsthand what it feels like to undergo and survive a transplant.

I know how difficult it is to make the decision to have a transplant, undergo the treatment, and get back to a normal life. I hope this book makes your experience a little easier.

Sue Stewart

Susan Stewart
Executive Director, BMT InfoNet

Chapter One
HISTORY OF TRANSPLANTATION

When I was first diagnosed with leukemia, I got very little encouragement from my local oncologist. Back then, bone marrow transplants weren't so common. He really tried to discourage me. He said 'A transplant is not for you. You might as well give up'. It felt pretty good to come home after my transplant, a survivor.

Jean, 15-year transplant survivor

Bone marrow, peripheral blood stem cell and umbilical cord blood transplantation are medical procedures used to treat people with diseases once thought incurable. Patients diagnosed with diseases such as leukemia, myelodysplastic syndrome (MDS), Hodgkin disease, non-Hodgkin lymphoma, multiple myeloma, a number of other blood and genetic disorders, some solid tumors and some autoimmune diseases may be a candidate for transplantation.

The technical name for bone marrow, peripheral blood stem cell and cord blood transplantation is hematopoietic stem cell transplantation.

Throughout this book, we will use the term blood stem cell transplant or stem cell transplant to refer to bone marrow, peripheral blood stem cell or cord blood transplants.

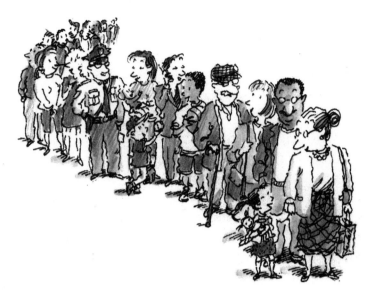

Types of Transplants

There are three types of transplant:

- allogeneic (al-o-je-náy-ik)
- syngeneic (sin-je-náy-ik)
- autologous (aw-tól-o-gus).

Patients with bone marrow disorders such as leukemia or myelodysplastic syndrome (MDS) typically receive an allogeneic transplant. In this procedure, the diseased bone marrow is destroyed by high-dose chemotherapy and/or radiation and replaced with a donor's blood stem cells.

Allogeneic transplants are the type of transplant discussed in this book.

Syngeneic transplantation is similar to allogeneic transplantation. The difference is that the donor is an identical twin, rather than another relative or an unrelated donor.

In an autologous transplant, your own stem cells are used for the transplant. Patients with diseases like multiple myeloma are usually treated with an autologous transplant. Autologous transplants are discussed in our book *Autologous Stem Cell Transplants: A Handbook for Patients*.

A Historical Perspective

The first serious attempts to transplant bone marrow into humans occurred in the late 1950s. Although several patients achieved a remission after transplant (there was no evidence of disease), most of them relapsed (the disease came back) shortly thereafter.

In the early 1960's, at least two successful transplants occurred using bone marrow donated by an identical twin – one in the U.S and another in China. Both patients were children diagnosed with severe aplastic anemia and were cured following their transplant.

The first successful transplant using bone marrow donated by a sibling who was **not** an identical twin took place in 1968. The patient was a baby boy who was born with an immune deficiency disease that had taken the life of all eleven male children born on his mother's side of the family. After two transplants, the child returned home and grew to be a healthy adult.

Similar successes were soon reported for patients with leukemia. By 1990, hundreds of transplant centers worldwide were performing bone marrow transplants.

Unrelated Donors

Unfortunately, many patients who could benefit from a bone marrow transplant could not undergo the procedure because they did not have a sibling with a matching marrow type. In 1973, two teams of researchers overcame this obstacle:

- The first, in England, successfully transplanted a 2-year-old child with a rare blood disorder called chronic granulomatous disease (CGD) using marrow donated by an unrelated person identified through a donor drive orchestrated by the child's mother. The patient is still alive today.

- Later that year, a team of doctors in New York completed a successful unrelated donor transplant for an infant born with severe combined immunodeficiency (SCID).

In the early 1980s, several local marrow donor registries sprang up throughout the United States. In 1986, the U.S. Congress created the National Marrow Donor Registry (now called the Be The

Match® Registry) to coordinate donor recruitment and facilitate more transplants with marrow from unrelated donors. Since then, more than 100,000 patients have received transplants with blood stem cells from an unrelated donor.

> The longest living transplant survivor is Nancy King McLain who underwent a bone marrow transplant with marrow from her twin sister, Bonnie, in 1963. Today, Nancy is a retired teacher who enjoys horseback riding, skating and skiing.
>
> "I love life every day because I know how close I came to losing it at such an early age," says Nancy.

Cord Blood Transplants

Despite a surge of volunteer bone marrow donors in the late 1980s and early 1990s, the number of people able to find an unrelated bone marrow donor remained small, compared to the need.

Researchers at Indiana University believed that cells in the discarded placenta and umbilical cord of newborn babies could be an alternate source of cells for transplant.

In 1988, that theory was put to the test. A five-year-old child in North Carolina was diagnosed with a blood disorder called Fanconi Anemia. Unable to find a matching bone marrow donor, his doctor proposed an experimental cord blood transplant with cells collected from the umbilical cord of his soon-to-be-born baby sister.

The transplant took place in Paris, France. After six months, the child was able to return home. Today he works at a cord blood bank where he counsels patients and potential cord blood donors.

Initially, cord blood transplants were only an option for children or small adults, due to the limited number of blood stem cells in each cord blood unit. Today, however, techniques such as combining two units of cord blood or manipulating the cord blood unit to increase the number of cells, are making cord blood transplantation a treatment option for large adults as well. The availability of cord blood has increased the number of patients who can benefit from an allogeneic transplant, especially those from diverse ethnic and racial backgrounds.

Peripheral Blood Stem Cell Transplants

In the late 1980s, researchers discovered that blood stem cells in the bone marrow could be moved to the bloodstream where they could be collected for transplant.

By the end of the 1990s, many medical centers were transplanting patients with blood stem cells collected from the bloodstream instead of, or in addition to, bone marrow. This procedure is called a peripheral blood stem cell transplant.

Reduced Intensity, Nonmyeloablative Transplants

It has been known for some time that the donor's white blood cells play a key role in destroying disease. A newer form of transplantation called nonmyeloablative or reduced intensity transplantation relies primarily on the disease-fighting power of the donor's immune system to kill the patient's disease.

There are fewer early side effects from this type of transplant since lower dosages of chemotherapy and/or radiation are given prior to transplant. However graft-versus-host disease (GVHD), a serious side effect of transplant, remains an issue.

Haploidentical Transplants

Haploidentical transplants, or half-matched transplants, are a newer form of transplant that has greatly increased the number of patients who can have a blood stem cell transplant. In this type of transplant, the donor can be a parent, child or sibling who is only half-matched with the patient.

Initially, haploidentical transplants resulted in a much higher incidence of relapse (the disease came back) and death compared to matched donor transplants. Patients also experienced a greater incidence of graft-versus-host disease.

Today, outcomes are often similar to those achieved using a fully matched donor.

A Look into the Future

Promising research is underway to improve on the results currently achieved with allogeneic transplantation. Many people with diseases once thought incurable are now leading productive and fulfilling lives, thanks to progress made in the field of blood stem cell transplantation.

Watch a video about the history of transplantation at

bmtinfonet.org/video/history-transplants

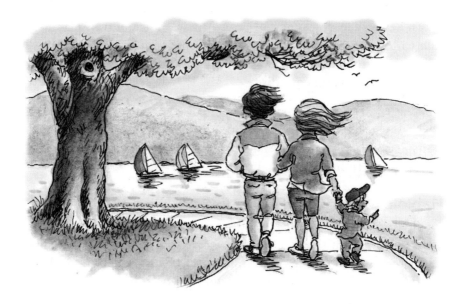

Chapter Two

AN INTRODUCTION TO TRANSPLANTATION

I still find it bizarre that I would be the one to get so sick. I was very physically active. I rode my bike 2,000 miles a year, swam about 100 miles, and was active in my children's lives. Cancer happens to people you read about in the newspaper. It doesn't strike an enormously healthy, happy and vital 39-year-old family man.

Mike, 11-year transplant survivor

This chapter will give you a broad overview of blood stem cell transplantation. The information can assist you in deciding whether or not to undergo a transplant, proceed with a decision you've already made, or understand the treatment that a loved one is undergoing. The remaining chapters of this book provide more detailed information about various aspects of blood stem cell transplantation.

What are Bone Marrow and Blood Stem Cells?

Bone marrow is a spongy tissue found inside bones. Bone marrow contains blood stem cells — special cells that generate most of the body's blood cells.

Blood stem cells produce:

- white blood cells (leukocytes) to fight infection

- red blood cells (erythrocytes) to carry oxygen to and remove waste products from organs and tissues
- platelets that enable blood to clot

Blood stem cells are different from the embryonic stem cells that are the topic of much public debate. Blood stem cells are collected from healthy donors or an umbilical cord, rather than from embryos that have not yet matured.

If you are considering a blood stem cell transplant, you may want to familiarize yourself with the different types of blood cells and their functions. During your treatment, the medical team will count and refer to these different blood cells frequently. For a detailed discussion of blood cells go to Appendix A, About Blood Cells, at the back of the book.

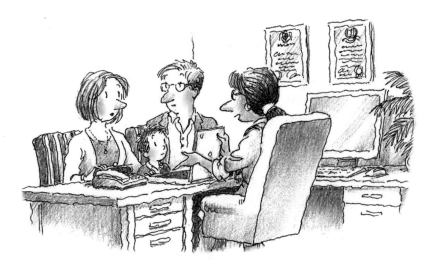

Why a Blood Stem Cell Transplant?

Sometimes the blood stem cells in bone marrow malfunction and begin producing too many defective or immature blood cells. The abnormal cells interfere with the production of normal blood cells and may invade other tissues.

Alternatively, the blood stem cells may produce too few blood cells. When either of these events occurs, a blood stem cell transplant may be the recommended treatment.

A blood stem cell transplant may also be a treatment option for you if you have an inherited disease such as certain immune deficiency diseases.

Source of Stem Cells

Since bone marrow contains the greatest concentration of blood stem cells, historically, most patients were transplanted with bone marrow. Most pediatric patients are still transplanted with bone marrow today.

However, it is now possible to move a large number of blood stem cells out of the bone marrow into the bloodstream where they can be collected and used instead of bone marrow. Transplants using stem cells collected from the bloodstream are called peripheral blood stem cell transplants.

Umbilical cord blood is also rich in blood stem cells. Although the quantity of blood stem cells in umbilical cord blood is small, it can also be used successfully in transplants.

Many factors such as your particular diagnosis, donor factors, risk of infection and risk of developing graft-versus-host disease will go into determining which stem cell source is best for you.

Who Can Undergo a Stem Cell Transplant?

To be a candidate for a blood stem cell transplant, you must have a suitable donor and be healthy enough to tolerate the transplant procedure.

When determining if you are a good candidate for transplant, your physician will consider your age, general physical condition, diagnosis, stage of the disease and prior treatment.

Tests of your heart, lungs, kidneys and other vital organs are performed prior to transplantation to ensure you can tolerate the procedure. These tests are later used as a baseline against which post-transplant tests can be compared. The pre-transplant tests are usually done during an outpatient visit.

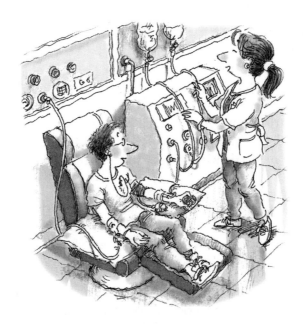

Who Can Be a Stem Cell Donor?

In order to be a suitable donor, genetic markers on the donor's blood cells must closely match yours. If the donor's cells are not a good match, they may perceive your organs and tissue as foreign material that should be destroyed. This condition is known as graft-versus-host disease (GVHD).

Alternatively, your immune system may destroy the donor's stem cells. This is called graft rejection.

If you have siblings who share the same biological parents, each has a 25 percent chance of being a suitable donor for you. If you don't have a matched sibling, you may be able to find a matched unrelated donor through the Be The Match® Registry, operated by the National Marrow Donor Program®. More than 5,000 transplants take place each year using blood stem cells provided by an unrelated donor or cord blood unit.

It may also be possible to use stem cells from your parent, child or a sibling who is only a partial match. This type of transplant is called a haploidentical transplant and is offered as a treatment option at many transplant centers in the U.S.

Preparative/Conditioning Regimen

Before the transplant can occur, your diseased marrow must be destroyed by high-dose chemotherapy or by a combination of high-dose chemotherapy and radiation. This phase of treatment is called the preparative or conditioning regimen.

The exact combination of high-dose chemotherapy and/or radiation varies according to the disease being treated and the protocol or preferred treatment plan of the transplant center. The preparative regimen usually lasts between four and ten days.

Most chemotherapy drugs are given through a thin flexible tube called a catheter or central venous line. The catheter is surgically implanted into a large vein in the chest, just above the heart. It allows the medical staff to give drugs and blood products to you painlessly, and to withdraw the many blood samples required during the course of treatment without inserting needles into your arms.

The catheter may be left in place for several months after transplant so that you can continue to have blood withdrawn and receive medications painlessly.

(For more on preparative regimens, see Chapter Nine, Preparative Regimen.)

The Transplant

One-to-three days after the preparative regimen, the transplant occurs.

- The donor's cells are infused into you through the catheter. The infusion typically takes 30 minutes to an hour to complete.

- You will be awake and may be lightly sedated during the transplant.

- You will be checked frequently for signs of fever, chills, hives and chest pains.

- You will not be in an operating room, as this is not surgery.

After the cells are infused, the days and weeks of waiting for the stem cells to begin producing healthy blood cells begin.

Engraftment

The two-to-three week period after the transplant is a critical time. The preparative regimen will have destroyed your stem cells, temporarily crippling your immune system. Until the donor's stem cells begin producing normal blood cells, you will be very susceptible to infection and excessive bleeding.

- You may receive drugs called growth factors to speed recovery of your blood counts.
- You will be given antibiotics and blood transfusions, as needed, to help prevent and fight infection.
- Platelet transfusions will help prevent bleeding.
- You may also take medications to reduce the risk of developing graft-versus-host disease.

Precautions will be taken to minimize your exposure to viruses and bacteria. Medical personnel will wash their hands with antiseptic soap and may wear gloves and/or a mask while visiting you. In addition, you may need to:

- wear a mask when leaving the clinic or the hospital room
- avoid foods that may contain harmful bacteria. (See Chapter Twelve, Nutrition for more details.)
- avoid young children, people who are sick and certain pets until your immune system is functioning normally.

If you undergo a reduced intensity transplant you are less likely to develop a severe infection during this period. (For more details on infection see Chapter 11, Infection.)

Daily blood samples will be taken to determine whether the stem cells have begun producing healthy blood cells. When blood counts begin to rise, some antibiotics and blood and platelet transfusions will generally no longer be required.

Once your stem cells are producing a sufficient number of healthy blood cells, you will be discharged from the hospital or outpatient center, provided no other complications have developed.

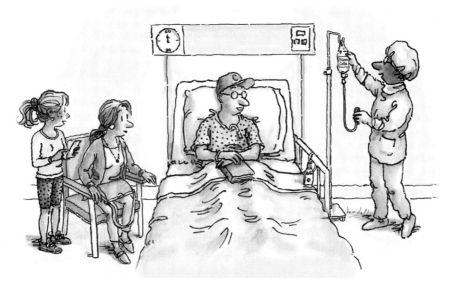

How Patients Feel During Treatment

A blood stem cell transplant is a physically and emotionally taxing procedure for both you and your family. You should seek as much help as possible to cope with the transplant experience.

After the preparative regimen, you will feel very tired, sick and weak. You may experience nausea, vomiting, fever and diarrhea. Activities like walking, sitting up in bed for long periods of time, reading books, talking on the phone, visiting with friends or even watching TV may require more energy than you have available.

Complications such as infection and bleeding can develop after transplant. Mouth sores may make eating and swallowing uncomfortable.

Temporary mental confusion, usually related to the medications, sometimes occurs. This can be quite frightening for you and loved ones who may not realize that it's usually temporary. The medical staff can help you deal with these problems.

Handling Emotional Stress

In addition to the physical discomfort, there is also emotional stress. You may find the emotional stress more problematic than the physical discomfort. Not only do you have to handle the fact that you have a life-threatening disease, but you may be fearful of the transplant procedure itself. While the transplant offers hope for a cure or longer life, there are no guarantees. Living with that uncertainty can be one of the biggest challenges people face long-term. Recognizing that there are things you do not control and focusing on the immediate things you do control can help.

You may also feel quite isolated. Special precautions taken to guard against infection during recovery make it difficult to interact normally with family and friends. Some friends and family members may not understand, or are poorly equipped to manage the gravity of the situation and the emotional trauma involved.

Remember that there are different ways that people can support you at different times or for different needs you have. Accepting different strengths of people around you can help you feel less disappointed in some family members or friends.

- One person might be there for all your emotional ups and downs but not have a clue when your family can use help with grocery shopping or other household chores.
- Another person may be good at shopping but not at helping you with the physical and emotional part of your journey.

Helplessness is a common feeling among transplant patients and can cause anger or resentment. It can be uncomfortable to rely totally on strangers for survival, no matter how competent they may be. You may also find it embarrassing to be dependent on others for help with basic daily functions such as using the bathroom.

Your lack of familiarity with the medical terms used to describe the transplant procedure can make you feel vulnerable and helpless. As the process becomes more familiar to you, however, you will likely feel less helpless.

Practice taking charge and directly asking for help with what you need. You may not be able to control everything, but it will feel good to exert some control over your situation.

The time spent waiting for blood counts to return to safe levels increases the emotional load. Recovery can be like a roller coaster ride: one day you may feel much better only to awake the next day feeling

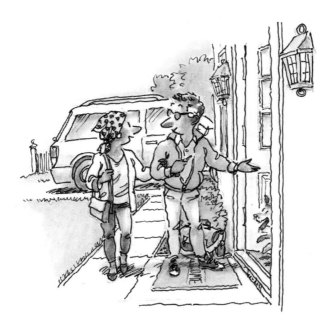

as sick as ever. (For more details see Chapter Seven, Emotional Challenges.)

First Year after Transplant

The length and nature of the recovery period varies from patient to patient. It may take a year or more before you are well enough to resume a normal routine and return to school or work.

It is best not to set unrealistic recovery goals or compare your progress to that of another patient. The length of the recovery period is not a good indication of whether or not you have been cured, or how long life has been extended. Some patients simply take longer to recover than others and can look forward to a long, healthy life.

You may develop an infection or other complications several weeks or months after transplant and need to be hospitalized for treatment. This can be discouraging.

It helps to keep in mind that these setbacks are common, and are usually temporary and reversible. Remind yourself that when you are back to being healthy, even weeks or months of frustration or setbacks will seem like a brief time. It will be well worth it to keep going even though in the moment it can be hard to tolerate.

Many patients develop graft-versus-host disease (GVHD) after transplant. Drugs used to manage GVHD can cause temporary weight gain, mood swings and other side effects that can make the recovery period more difficult. (For more details see Chapter Ten, Graft-versus-Host Disease.)

Life during the first year after transplant can be both exhilarating and worrisome. On the one hand, it is exciting to be alive after being so close to death. Some survivors find their quality of life improves after transplant.

Nonetheless, you will likely worry that the disease will come back. It can be many months before one full day passes when you don't think about the disease or transplant experience. It may take several years before you can allow yourself to believe you have truly been cured. Even though it can seem like a long process, allow yourself to feel good about what you have accomplished along the way. (For a discussion of long-term concerns after transplant see Chapter Fifteen, Planning for Survivorship.)

Is It Worth It?

Many survivors report that their quality of life after transplant is as good or better than before transplant. While transplants are not always successful, and complications can create a "new normal" for some, stem cell transplants have cured or prolonged the lives of thousands of people. These survivors are grateful to have been given a new lease on life.

> "Currently, I'm 14 months post-transplant. I celebrated my one-year anniversary by climbing a mountain in Colorado and getting second row seats for a Jimmy Buffet concert. Lots of people celebrated with me and gave me inspirational messages, gifts and support. My favorite gift was from my doctor — an interpretation of my bone marrow biopsy. The interpretation pretty much describes my life today. Normal."

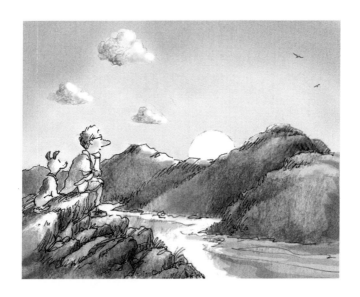

To learn more visit our website at:

bmtinfonet.org/transplant-basics

Chapter Three

CHOOSING A TRANSPLANT CENTER

Was I scared? I was scared as a rabbit in winter. But I kept thinking, 'there's light at the end of the tunnel and I'm not ready to give up'. I remember the day they put me in the hospital. My 13-year-old son said 'I'm wrapping an invisible rope around you, mom. Slowly but surely I'm going to tug on it until I get you back home again'. That was the most wonderful thing in the world. I'll never forget that he said that.

Maralyn, 19-year transplant survivor

In the early days of transplantation, allogeneic stem cell transplants were offered by only a handful of medical centers worldwide. Today more than 200 hospitals perform allogeneic transplants in the U.S. alone. How do you decide which medical center is best for you?

Depending on your insurance coverage, the choice may be wide open or very limited. Many U.S. insurers negotiate contracts with a handful of transplant centers and require their plan enrollees to be treated at these centers. Although such plans limit your choices, the designated medical centers are usually major institutions with a highly experienced transplant team that provides excellent care.

Your particular disease may limit the number of centers available for consideration. For example, while many centers perform transplants for patients with leukemia, fewer offer the treatment for patients with some immune deficiency diseases or inherited blood disorders.

Your oncologist or hematologist may recommend a particular center for treatment. The recommendation may be based on a number of obvious factors like the transplant team's experience and reputation. Other less obvious factors may include the relationship your doctor has with the transplant team, and his or her prior experience getting information from the transplant center when you return home for follow-up care. Ask why your doctor recommends one center over another, and don't hesitate to explore other transplant centers as well.

BMT InfoNet maintains a list of hospitals that perform allogeneic transplants in the U.S. and Canada which includes information on the number of transplants performed, diseases treated, accreditation and contact information. Go to bmtinfonet.org/transplantcenters or phone 888-597-7674. Be The Match® also maintains a list of transplant centers.

If you are free to choose between different centers, there are several factors you'll want to consider.

Accreditation

The Foundation for Accreditation of Cellular Therapy (FACT) is an organization that inspects transplant programs and accredits those that meet the FACT standards. Although transplant centers are not required to seek FACT accreditation, FACT accreditation is a sign that the program has passed a rigorous inspection and is considered by experts in the field to be a quality transplant program. Go to factwebsite.org to learn which programs are FACT accredited.

The Transplant Team

When considering a transplant center, focus first on the transplant team — the doctors, nurses, radiologists, pharmacists and other support staff who will be involved in your care. The more training and experience they have in dealing with transplant patients, the better they will be able to respond to problems.

Doctors

The transplant program director should be a licensed physician with board certification in hematology, medical oncology, immu-

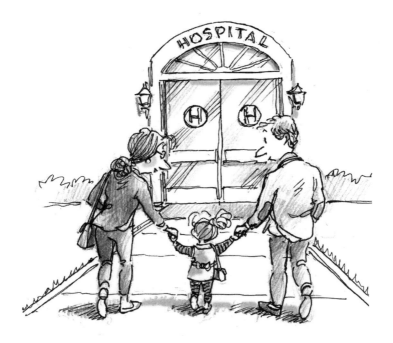

nology and/or pediatric hematology/oncology. The other transplant physicians who will be involved in your care should also be licensed and board certified in one of those specialties.

Questions to ask about the doctors include:

- How much training or experience do the transplant doctors have in caring for transplant patients?

- Will a transplant physician be on call 24/7 to handle emergencies and answer questions?

- If you have a pre-existing medical condition that may complicate your treatment, such as a heart or lung problem, how much experience do the doctors have in handling patients with similar problems?

- Does the transplant team have around-the-clock access to other licensed specialists who may need to be involved in your care, such as doctors who are board certified in surgery, pulmonary medicine, intensive care, gastroenterology, nephrology, infectious diseases, cardiology, pathology, psychiatry and radiation therapy?

Nurses

A highly-trained, experienced team of nurses is a critical component of a good transplant program. It's the nurses who spend the most time with patients. They must be able to quickly identify problems and respond appropriately.

Questions to ask about the nursing staff include:

- How many registered nurses will be involved in your care?
- How many have been trained and certified in hematology/oncology?
- How much experience have they had caring for transplant patients?
- What is the nurse-to-patient ratio?
- Do the nurses receive ongoing education about caring for transplant patients?

Psychosocial Support Services

Undergoing a blood stem cell transplant is not only physically difficult but emotionally taxing as well. You may find the emotional strain more difficult to handle than the physical discomfort.

Even if you have never before sought counseling, you may need the help of a psychiatrist, psychologist, social worker or religious counselor to help you cope with the transplant experience. Remember that when a journey is entirely unfamiliar and frightening, it helps to have someone with you who knows the road. This is true not only for your physical experiences but also for your emotional experiences.

Psychosocial support services offered by transplant centers vary considerably. Ask whether support is routinely provided or if it is available upon request. Find out what other programs are available to help you and your family members cope emotionally, such as support groups, music therapy or massage therapy.

Pediatric Patients

If the transplant patient is a child, find out whether the doctors, nurses and support staff have training and experience in treating pediatric patients. Children are not just small adults. Their growing bodies may react differently to drugs, and their emotional needs are different as well.

Some transplant centers specialize in treating only pediatric patients, while others treat both children and adults — sometimes with the same staff. If the center you're considering does not limit its practice to pediatric patients, be sure that the team members, as well as consulting specialists, are experienced in caring for pediatric patients.

Some centers have strict guidelines about how long the parent can remain with a hospitalized child and require parents to leave in the evening. Others will allow parents to remain overnight if they wish. Make sure you're comfortable with the center's guidelines on this matter.

Ask what sort of age-appropriate activities and counseling will be provided to your child during treatment, particularly if your child is a teen. Inquire about the center's philosophy on providing pain medication for uncomfortable procedures such as bone marrow aspirates. Can your child bring favorite toys, clothes, etc. to his or her hospital room?

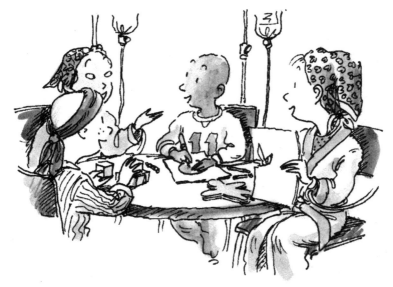

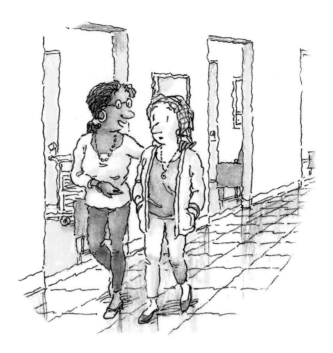

Support for Family Caregivers

Most transplant programs require that you have a caregiver who can be with you at the hospital, and who is available to care for you 24/7 once you return home.

Ask what sort of support systems are in place to help your caregivers.

- Find out what kind of training caregivers will receive.

- Ask whether your caregiver will have access to volunteers who can help with routine daily tasks, such as shopping or laundry, while your caregiver is with you, especially if the transplant is taking place out of town.

- Ask what kind of psychosocial support is available for your caregiver.

Number of Transplants Performed

Although the training and experience of the transplant team members are the most important factors to evaluate, the number of transplants performed by a center can often give you a rough idea of the team's experience. Keep in mind, however, that transplant teams and team members frequently relocate to different hospitals. Fifty transplants may have been performed at a center during the past two years, but not necessarily by the team that will care for you now.

You can find out how many transplants have been performed at a center by inquiring at the center directly or at bmtinfonet.org/transplantcenters or by calling BMT InfoNet at 888-597-7674.

Treatment Plans

The treatment plan or 'protocol' for a particular disease can vary from center to center. The type and dosage of chemotherapy drugs may differ. Some centers may be testing new methods of handling transplant complications. Others may be investigating novel ways to prevent relapse.

The risks associated with various treatment plans may differ as well. Ask what is known about the effectiveness and risks associated with the particular protocol suggested for you. Find out what will be done to manage the complications and satisfy yourself that the center has the experience necessary to spot and quickly treat problems when they arise.

Ask the doctor to be as specific as possible in describing how patients that are similar to you (e.g., same age, stage of disease and medical problems) have fared. Keep in mind, however, that such data may not be available for newer treatment plans.

Success Rates

The question asked most often by patients is 'Which transplant center has the best success rate?'

A 'successful transplant' can be defined in different ways. It may mean that the stem cells engrafted and the patient did not die of complications while in the hospital or clinic. Alternatively, 'successful transplant' may mean that the patient lived one, three, five years or more without a recurrence of the disease. When discussing success rates with transplant centers, be sure you understand how they are defining the term.

Transplant teams may use the terms 'event-free survival' (EFS) or 'disease-free survival' (DFS) when discussing their success rate. Although they sound similar, each statistic measures success differently.

Event-free survival tells you how many patients, out of all that were transplanted, are alive and disease-free a specific number of years after transplant. If 100 patients were transplanted and 40 are still alive and disease-free three years after transplant, the three year event-free survival is 40 percent (40 patients divided by 100 patients).

Disease-free survival, on the other hand, focuses only on the patients who were *in remission* after transplant. In other words, if only 50 out of 100 patients were in remission after their transplant, and 40 of those 50 were still alive and disease-free three years later, the disease-free survival would be 80% (40 patients divided by 50 patients).

On first glance, it might look like the transplant center with the 80% disease-free survival had more successful transplants than the center with a 40 percent event-free survival but, in fact, the success rates were similar. Both had 40 out of 100 survivors alive and disease-free three years after transplant.

Don't compare event-free survival rates at one center to disease-free survival rates at another. It's like comparing apples to oranges. Ask for both figures, and be sure they are for a comparable group of patients followed over a comparable length of time.

Many factors influence a center's success rate. For example, a hospital that accepts only prime candidates for transplant — young people, those in an early stage of their disease, and those who have responded well to prior treatment— may report better success rates than centers who accept older or sicker patients.

When asking about success rates, be sure the figure you're given is for:

- transplants for patients who had the the same treatment plan that is proposed for you
- patients who were similar to you in age, diagnosis and other health problems
- patients treated at the transplant center you care considering, rather than another transplant center

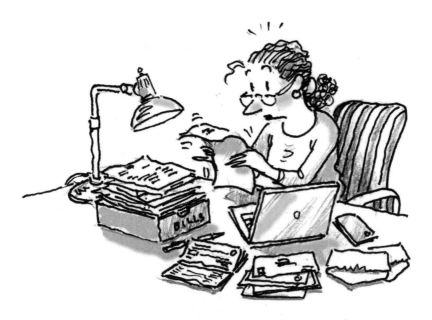

Success rates from other centers may be better or worse than success rates achievable at the center you're considering.

Be The Match® provides data on one-year survival rates at U.S. transplant centers. Go to bmtinfonet.org/choosing-transplant-center for a link to this data.

Finances

Allogeneic transplants are very costly even if insurance is paying for all or most of the procedure. In addition to medical expenses, families may incur large travel, lodging and meal expenses, particularly if the patient is being treated out of town. You may have large insurance co-pays and deductibles. If a caregiver must take time off from work to be with the patient, this can add to the financial burden.

Talk to the social worker at the transplant center to find out what sort of assistance is available to help defray these expenses. Some centers have special arrangements with local hotels or dormitories to house patients and family members at low or no cost. Others can help you apply for financial assistance.

If convincing your insurance company to pay for the transplant is a problem, find out what sort of help the center will provide. Most are well prepared to handle insurance company inquiries and are experienced in persuading insurers to pay for your care. Some are not. Ask if the transplant team will help you appeal an insurer's denial of coverage should that occur. (For more on insurance, see Chapter Six, Insurance and Fundraising.)

If insurance refuses to pay for your treatment, ask what sort of alternative financing arrangement the center is willing to make with you. Most centers will refuse to provide treatment unless insurance pre-approves payment or the family makes a hefty down payment.

Charges for a blood stem cell transplant vary considerably from center to center. A center may not be able to quote an exact price for your treatment, since the cost of your care will depend on how long you need to be hospitalized and any special treatment needs. If one is available, ask to speak to a transplant financial counselor who may be able to provide you more detailed information about out-of-pocket costs.

Long-Term Follow-Up

After you leave the transplant center, your care will eventually be turned over to your local doctor, ideally a specialist like an oncologist or hematologist. Since most doctors have not received specific training in the care of transplant patients, it's important that the transplant center staff be accessible to both you and your doctor to handle questions and provide guidance about your care.

Find out whether the transplant center will keep your local doctor updated on your treatment and progress. Ask if you and your doctor will receive written instructions about follow-up care. You should both feel comfortable contacting your transplant center directly to discuss questions and concerns.

Guidelines for long-term follow-up care of blood stem cell transplant patients have been published by the American Society for Transplantation and Cellular Therapy (ASTCT), the Center for International Blood and Marrow Transplant Research (CIBMTR) and the European Group for Blood and Marrow Transplantation (EBMT). Access these guidelines through the BMT InfoNet website at bmtinfonet.org/long-term-health-guidelines or phone 888-597-7674.

Many transplant centers strongly encourage patients to return to the center annually, at least for the first few years, for follow-up care.

The Bottom Line

Happily, there are many excellent transplant programs that provide top quality medical care. For most patients, no one program will clearly be superior. Rather, you and your doctor will be able to choose among a number of highly qualified transplant programs.

Keep in mind that you and your family are important members of the transplant team. It's important that you're comfortable with the staff at the center where you'll be treated, and that worries about issues such as insurance, allowing your spouse to continue working and having family members well cared for are kept to a minimum. Working with your doctor, you should be able to identify the programs that best suit your family's medical, financial and emotional needs.

To learn more about transplant centers go to our website at:

bmtinfonet.org/transplantcenters

Chapter Four
FINDING A DONOR

My younger brother, Gary, was my donor. We were always close, but not as close as we are now. We feel like we're part of each other. I wouldn't have a life to live if it weren't for him.

Melinda, one-year transplant survivor

It would be wonderful if patients who need a stem cell transplant could ask any willing relative or friend to be their donor. Unfortunately, it's not that simple. Both patient and donor must have a similar tissue type in order for the transplant to be successful.

Genetic markers on the surface of your cells define your tissue type. Since these markers are inherited from parents, your siblings are much more likely to have the same tissue type than another relative. Each sibling has a 25 percent chance of being a perfect match for their brother or sister.

A newer type of transplant, called haploidentical transplant, makes it possible for other family members who are only a half-match for the patient to be a donor. These potential donors include parents and children of the patient as well as some siblings who are not a perfect match.

If no related donor is available, a search for an unrelated donor can be initiated.

What Are They Matching?

On the surface of your cells lie sets of proteins. Like a fingerprint, these proteins enable your immune system to distinguish between cells that belong in your body and cells that do not. If your immune system cells encounter a cell with the wrong fingerprint, they orchestrate an immune system attack to destroy it.

Several different proteins on the surface of white blood cells, called human leukocyte antigens (HLA), play an important role in stem cell transplantation. These HLA markers are referred to as HLA-A, HLA-B, HLA-C, HLA-DR, HLA-DP and HLA-DQ. You inherit one set of these HLA markers from your mother and another from your father.

Research has shown that patients whose HLA type closely matches that of the donor have a better outcome after transplant.

Each transplant center has its own criteria for an acceptable match, which can vary depending on the type of transplant you are having (related versus unrelated) and the type of blood stem cell being used (stem cells collected from the bloodstream verses bone marrow versus cord blood).

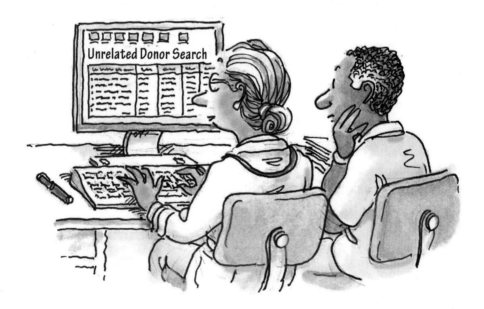

Unrelated Donor Search

In the United States, the Be The Match® Registry operated by the National Marrow Donor Program® coordinates the recruitment of unrelated donors. More than 35 million potential donors worldwide can be accessed through the Be The Match Registry. The registry includes both adult donors and cord blood units.

- Your doctor can do a preliminary search of the Be The Match Registry to assess the likelihood of finding a donor for you.

- If potential donors are identified in the preliminary search, the transplant center may then request a formal search.

- Promising looking donors will be contacted and additional tests will be done to confirm the person is, indeed, a good match.

Once the best donor is identified, he or she will receive extensive counseling by a Be The Match representative before giving final consent to donate. Potential donors undergo a complete medical evaluation to ensure they are healthy enough to donate and don't have any medical problems that could pose a risk to you.

> Often, a perfectly matched donor cannot be found immediately. In may take several months or longer to identify a suitable donor. Some patients will be advised to wait for a better matching donor, while others may need to proceed to transplant with a less than perfectly matched donor or choose a different treatment option such as a haploidentical transplant.

Cord Blood Transplants

A transplant using blood stem cells from an umbilical cord may be an option for you and is sometimes the preferred option. Cord blood units do not need to match your HLA-type as closely as bone marrow or peripheral blood stem cells from an adult donor. They can also be made available more quickly for transplant, since they have already been collected and stored for later use.

If More Than One Donor is Found

If more than one matched donor is available, several other factors will help determine the most suitable donor.

- Younger donors are usually preferred over older donors.
- Donors who have not been exposed to a common virus called cytomegalovirus (CMV) are preferable if you too have not been exposed to CMV.
- Some studies suggest that gender is important. Male patients transplanted with female stem cells appear to have a higher risk of developing chronic GVHD.

Working together with your transplant physician, you should be able to identify the best donor for you.

To find more about searching for a donor go to our website at:

bmtinfonet.org/finding-blood-stem-cell-donor

Chapter Five

BEING A DONOR

You feel so helpless when someone you love needs a transplant. I was joyous when I learned I might be able to save my sister's life by being a donor. Still, I worried that if the transplant failed it would be my fault. I knew that wasn't rational, but I couldn't help feeling that way. I prayed a lot and told myself I was giving my sister my best shot.

Linda, donor for seven-year transplant survivor

Each year thousands of people donate bone marrow or stem cells collected from the bloodstream, or their baby's discarded umbilical cord blood to save a life. Some do so for a loved one. Others offer this gift to someone they don't even know.

Although the opportunity to save a life is exciting, being a donor can also be emotionally challenging. Often, families are so focused on the needs of the patient that the donor's questions and concerns are overlooked.

This chapter will explain the procedure used to collect bone marrow and blood stem cells from donors. It will also discuss how donating marrow or stem cells may impact your health and the emotional challenges you may face.

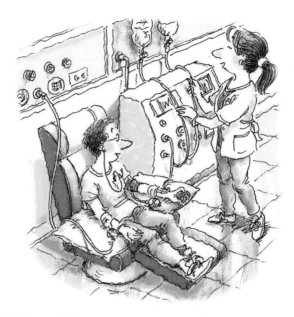

Stem Cell Harvest

If you are asked to provide stem cells collected from the bloodstream, the procedure is called a peripheral blood stem cell harvest. A stem cell harvest is not a surgical procedure and is usually performed in an outpatient clinic.

Prior to the harvest, you will be given injections of a drug called filgrastim (Neupogen®), or a drug similar to it, over a four-to-five-day period. Filgrastim is a man-made protein that is similar to a protein normally found in the body. The filgrastim helps move stem cells out of the bone marrow into the bloodstream where they can easily be collected.

When it is time to collect the stem cells, you will sit in a comfortable chair.

- A needle connected to flexible tubing will be inserted into a vein in each arm.

- Blood will be withdrawn from one arm and passed through a machine that separates out the stem cells.

- The rest of the blood will be returned to you through flexible tubing that is connected to the needle that was inserted in your other arm.

- If you have small arm veins, stem cells can be collected through special flexible tubing that is inserted into a large vein near the groin or under the collarbone.

Depending on the number of stem cells collected during each session, it may take two days, and in some cases three to five days, to collect enough stem cells for transplantation.

Some donors feel lightheaded, cold or numb around the lips during the collection. Others experience cramping in their hands which is caused by a blood-thinning agent used during the procedure that reduces the level of calcium in the blood. The cramping usually resolves after treatment with calcium supplements. Other possible short-term side effects include bone pain, headache, fatigue and nausea.

Bone Marrow Harvest

You may be asked to donate bone marrow, instead of peripheral blood stem cells. The procedure used to collect bone marrow from a donor is called a bone marrow harvest. It is a surgical procedure that takes place in the hospital operating room.

While you are under anesthesia, a needle will be inserted into your rear hip bone where a large quantity of bone marrow is located. The bone marrow, a thick red liquid, will be extracted with a needle and syringe.

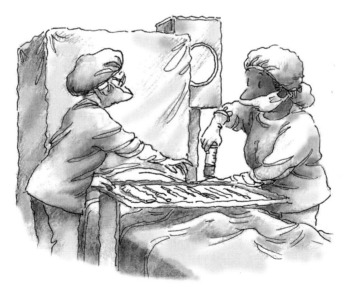

Several skin punctures on each hip and multiple bone punctures will be required to extract sufficient bone marrow for transplantation. There are no surgical incisions or stitches involved, only skin punctures where the needle was inserted, which will be covered with a sterile bandage.

The amount of bone marrow harvested depends on the size of the patient and the concentration of stem cells in your marrow. Usually, one-to-two quarts of marrow and blood are harvested. While this may sound like a lot, your body can usually replace it in four weeks.

When the anesthesia wears off, you may feel some discomfort at the harvest site. The pain will be similar to that associated with a hard fall on the ice and can usually be controlled with acetaminophen. Most donors can resume normal activities in a few days although activities such as climbing stairs or sitting in one place for a long period of time may be uncomfortable for a week or two.

Impact on Your Health

In most cases, the medical procedure used to collect bone marrow or peripheral blood stem cells will have a minimal, short-term impact on your health. However, as with all medical procedures, there is a small chance that you may experience side effects that are more severe.

Before you agree to be a donor, you will need a physical exam to determine whether donating is safe for you. Be sure to share with the doctor your complete medical history including illnesses and surgeries you have had in the past, even if you don't think they are important, as well as any current health conditions.

Some donors are more comfortable having a different doctor than the patient's doctor conduct the exam and interview. This can ease concerns that the doctor will consider the patient's health more important than the donor's. If this is not the standard operating procedure at the hospital where your loved one is being treated, don't hesitate to request an independent doctor if it will make you feel more comfortable.

Be sure to tell the doctor if any of the following conditions apply to you:

- AIDS/HIV
- severe arthritis, such as rheumatoid arthritis
- severe asthma
- autoimmune disease such as multiple sclerosis, systemic lupus, chronic fatigue syndrome or fibromyalgia
- back, hip, neck or spinal problems or surgeries
- bleeding problems such as hemophilia, aplastic anemia or a history of more than one deep vein blood clot
- breathing problems such as chronic obstructive pulmonary disease, emphysema, sleep apnea or cystic fibrosis
- a history of cancer
- a history of depression or other mental health problems
- diabetes
- epilepsy
- heart disease, heart attacks or a history of heart surgery

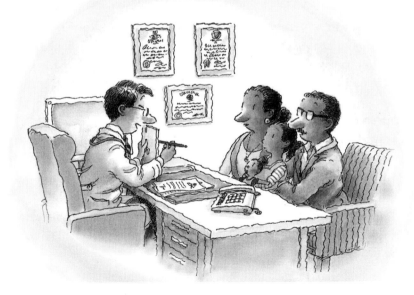

- hepatitis or possible exposure to hepatitis
- history of jaundice caused by mononucleosis or cytomegalovirus (CMV)
- kidney problems
- liver disease such as hepatitis, cirrhosis or Wilson's disease
- lyme disease
- prior organ or tissue transplant recipient
- pregnancy
- tuberculosis
- problems with general or regional anesthesia

Many of these conditions do not necessarily exclude you from being a donor but should be thoroughly discussed with the doctor.

Ask Your Questions

It is common for donors to be reluctant to ask the medical team many questions about being a donor. Everyone is focused on helping the transplant recipient get well, and donors sometimes feel selfish asking questions about their own health or seeking counseling if they have doubts or worries.

It's important to remember that you are a patient too. Your health and well-being are every bit as important as that of the patient. You are entitled to have your questions and concerns thoroughly addressed. If an answer is unclear, keep asking until you understand it.

Who Pays for All This?

If you are donating marrow or stem cells to an unrelated person, your medical expenses will be covered by the patient. If you are donating cells to a relative, the patient's insurance typically covers this expense. However, this is not always the case. The donor's health insurance rarely covers these expenses. The transplant center needs to work out arrangements with the patient on how these costs will be covered.

Other financial issues to consider:

- Some donors need to take time off work for the physical exam which can result in lost pay.
- The actual collection of the bone marrow or peripheral blood stem cells from the donor may require additional time off work.
- If the donor is asked to travel out of town in order to donate, this too will require time off work.

Lost pay and travel expenses are typically not covered by the patient's insurance.

Explore Possible Outcomes

The likelihood of long-term success will depends on the patient's diagnosis, stage of disease, age, general health and prior treatments. Problems that can arise after transplant such as infection, organ damage or graft-versus-host disease can also impact survival. In some cases, the disease will come back several months or years after transplant.

> A very important question that donors often neglect to ask is 'Will I save my relative's life if I donate my marrow or stem cells?'
>
> The answer is maybe. If you have been selected as the best possible donor, you are giving your loved one a second chance at life. Even if you are a perfect match, there are many other factors that will determine whether the transplant is successful.

It's best to have a frank discussion with the doctor evaluating you as a potential donor about the possible outcomes of the transplant. Many donors assume that a cure is guaranteed if they donate their stem cells and are shocked if the patient develops serious complications or dies. Preparing yourself for all possible outcomes can help you cope if problems arise.

Emotional Challenges

Although it can be exciting to have the opportunity to give a loved one a second chance at life, it can be stressful as well.

- Many donors wonder what they can do to make their stem cells better.
- Some worry that if the transplant is not successful it will be their fault.

There is nothing you can do to make your stem cells stronger or better. Eating right, getting enough sleep, and making sure you are healthy enough to donate your bone marrow or peripheral blood stem cells when the time comes are the most important things you can do.

Even though many factors that determine the success of a transplant are beyond the donor's control, donors still often feel that they are responsible for the outcome. This can be a heavy emotional burden.

It can help to discuss your feelings with a counselor or with another person who has been a donor for a loved one.

- Your hospital may have social workers who can help you think through these concerns.
- BMT InfoNet's Caring Connections Program can put you in touch with other people who have been donors. You can request a Caring Connection by phoning BMT InfoNet at 888-597-7674 or online at bmtinfonet.org/caring-connection.

Don't ignore your feelings. Feeling nervous, scared, responsible for the outcome or unsure about whether you want to donate is normal. Talking about these feelings with others is important.

What if I Don't Want to Be a Donor?

Sometimes a person prefers not to be a donor. You may be concerned about your own health, feel pressure from a spouse not to donate, or have a medical condition which would disqualify you as a donor that you don't want to disclose to other family members.

If you are a reluctant donor, discuss your concerns frankly and confidentially with the transplant doctor assigned to you. Ask if the patient has other options if you choose not to be a donor.

The doctor should be able to inform the patient that you are not a possible donor without disclosing the reason why.

Many Different Outcomes

There is no way of predicting with certainty whether a transplant will succeed or fail. One thing is certain, however: you, the donor, are not responsible for the outcome. You've done your best by donating your marrow or peripheral blood stem cells. The many other factors that contribute to the success of a transplant are beyond your control.

Be cautiously optimistic when donating marrow or stem cells. Hope for the best but prepare for setbacks. With luck, your loved one will have many more years of life.

To learn more go to our website at:

bmtinfonet.org/being-related-donor or

bmtinfonet.org/being-unrelated-donor

Chapter Six
INSURANCE AND FUNDRAISING

Our insurance company said a double cord blood transplant was experimental and would not approve it. During an unbelievably stressful week, we contacted an attorney, looked into private pay options and asked the hospital how they could help. I don't know whether it was the letters from our transplant center and our attorney, or calls from us and my employer that did it, but a week later they changed their mind and agreed to pay for the transplant.

Julie, mother of five-year transplant survivor

Most transplant centers are skilled at providing insurers with the documentation they need to authorize coverage of a blood stem cell transplant. Fortunately, many patients have no difficulty persuading their insurer to pay for their transplant.

However, if you have difficulty with your insurance company, read on. The information in this section will help you understand how insurance companies make decisions, how you can appeal those decisions, when to enlist the help of an experienced attorney and what other funding options exist.

Insurance

A blood stem cell transplant is a very expensive medical procedure. Depending on the transplant center, the length of time you must be hospitalized, and complications that arise, the treatment can cost hundreds of thousands of dollars. It is therefore not surprising that most insurance companies are cautious when reviewing requests to approve this treatment.

The best way to minimize insurance problems is to start early. Since life gets more hectic if an insurance denial comes at the last minute, it's important that you and the transplant center take a few steps at the outset.

Plan Ahead

As soon as possible, ask the insurer to pre-approve the treatment. The transplant center, not you, should contact your insurer early in the planning process so that the company can review the request and resolve questions.

Gather all your insurance information early on. Get the latest copy of your full plan booklet (not the summary booklet usually given to plan participants), as well as copies of any other health insurance policies under which you are insured. If you later need to consult with an attorney, he or she will need all these documents to determine whether the insurer is legally required to cover the treatment under the terms of the contract.

Submit Complete Information

Most transplant centers send an information package to the insurer that includes a letter from the treating physician, as well as studies and articles supporting the recommended procedure. It's important that insurers get this information early on, and that it is complete and up-to-date. The letter from the doctor should stress that the treatment is the best available therapy for you, is safe and effective, and is widely accepted by the medical community. Articles and letters of support that explain why the treatment plan is appropriate should be current.

If Coverage is Denied

If your insurance company denies coverage of your medical treatment, it may be possible to reverse that decision.

Usually when insurers deny coverage for a blood stem cell transplant, they rely on language in the insurance contract that excludes

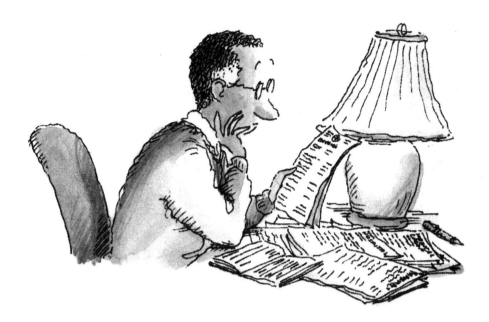

payment for experimental or investigational treatments. What insurers or doctors may consider experimental, however, can be quite different from the legal interpretation of experimental.

It's wise to consult an attorney who is experienced in this field of law to determine whether or not you may be able to successfully reverse a denial of coverage. Your letter of appeal should not be drafted by the attorney who helped you with your house closing or divorce. You need an attorney who is just as experienced in this field of law as your doctor is in this field of medicine.

Your transplant center may have the name of an attorney who successfully helped patients in the past. If not, you can contact BMT InfoNet at 888-597-7674 for a referral to an attorney who can help you.

Appealing a Denial of Coverage

The majority of insurance plans are governed by ERISA, a federal law that requires you to take steps within certain time frames if insurance coverage is denied. In most cases, you must first appeal your denial of coverage with the insurer before proceeding to a court appeal.

What you put in the letter of appeal will determine your rights later, should you have to go to court. Accordingly, you should keep the following points in mind.

1. In most cases, you are required to appeal a denial of coverage within 60 days or you lose all further rights of appeal. Some people are turned down at the last moment and go forward with treatment, figuring they'll deal with the insurance problem later on. When they do get around to filing an appeal, it is too late.

2. You and your doctor should include all evidence supporting the appropriateness of the therapy when you file the appeal. In most cases, if you later have to go to court to appeal an insurer's denial of coverage, the issue will be whether or not the insurer made an appropriate decision in light of the evidence it earlier received from your doctor

3. The appeal letter should clearly state why the procedure is appropriate for the treatment of your disease. It should identify all doctors the insurer should contact, list any favorable second opinions you received, and include instructions on how to contact doctors rendering these favorable opinions, should that be necessary.

Triage Cancer is an organization that provides a wealth of information about insurance benefits and your rights as an insurance consumer. Go to triagecancer.org.

Viatical Settlements and Accelerated Benefits

In the event that insurance does not cover some or all of the costs associated with a transplant and it becomes necessary to secure funding elsewhere, there are several options to consider.

Life insurance was once considered a source of funds only after a person died. But today, other options may be available for owners of life insurance who are terminally or chronically ill — viatical settlements and accelerated benefits. Both provide cash benefits while the policyholder is still alive. These benefits may be wholly or partially exempt from federal taxes.

Viatical Settlements

Viatical settlements appeared in the 1980s in reaction to the AIDS crisis. Brokers offered to purchase life insurance policies at a discount from terminally ill patients. Patients were free to use the money for medical expenses, or any other purpose.

Soon an industry arose with good and bad results. Patients who truly needed cash had a new source of funds. However, some received far less than the true value of their policy. Today, viatical settlements typically pay the patient 50-85% of the face value of the policy.

Accelerated Benefits

Some life insurance policies have a specific accelerated benefits option. Older policies may offer it on a case by case basis.

Many plans offer up to 75 percent of your benefit now, with the balance reserved as a true death benefit. There is usually an interest or transaction fee charged for taking an accelerated benefit.

The advantages of taking accelerated benefits rather than selling a policy to a viatical settlement provider are two-fold:

- It is often less costly to take accelerated benefits.
- You have the advantage of working with someone you know and trust.

A disadvantage is that the insurance company may restrict the amount of benefits you can accelerate or put restrictions on how you use the funds.

Is It Right for Me?

If you are considering a viatical settlement or accelerating your life insurance benefits, the following points should be considered:

1. Is there really a need for the money?

   Funds you withdraw now will not be available to pay for expenses they were originally intended to cover such as education and living expenses of your survivors. Do you really need the funds?

2. How will a viatical settlement or receipt of accelerated benefits affect your overall financial picture?

   An infusion of cash from a viatical settlement or accelerated benefits may affect your entitlement to public benefits, treatment of estate taxes and how your creditors view you. Some creditors may look to your viatical settlement funds as a ready source of payment. They may be less willing to enter into payment plans and may demand immediate payment.

   Check with a social worker or benefits counselor to determine the settlement's effect on benefits such as disability or Medicaid. Speak with your accountant or attorney to determine what the tax and estate consequences will be.

3. Does your insurance policy provide accelerated benefits?

   Before entering into a viatical settlement, check to see if your life insurance plan offers an accelerated benefits option. Accelerated benefits can be cheaper and easier than a viatical settlement because it is already part of your policy.

4. Get the best deal.

   Some viatical settlements offer you as little as 30 percent of the total life insurance proceeds. On a $300,000 life insurance policy, that would be $90,000 to the insured and $210,000 to the viatical settlement company. The amount is often dependent on life expectancy.

Other Fundraising Options

A number of organizations provide financial support for some of the costs associated or help patients conduct fundraisers. For a listing of these organizations, visit BMT InfoNet's online Resource Directory at bmtinfonet.org/resource-directory or phone 888-597-7674.

To learn more go to our website at:

bmtinfonet.org/insurance-and-financial-issues

Chapter Seven
EMOTIONAL CHALLENGES

There weren't any support groups for transplant patients in my area. If there had been a support group, I would have attended, because when they first tell you about the transplant and you start reading up on the subject, it can scare the heck out of you.

Dwight, 13-year transplant survivor

Stem cell transplantation provides hope for many patients diagnosed with diseases that were once thought incurable. This hope sustains patients and their families through the difficult period of treatment and recovery.

Nonetheless, contemplating a transplant, undergoing the procedure and coping with the recovery process is a trying experience for patients, families and friends.

This chapter will discuss the fears and emotions that are typical during transplant. Throughout the chapter, you will find direct quotations from people who survived their transplant and have offered to share their insights.

Coping With the News

When facing the prospect of a transplant, the news can be devastating.

- You may have not yet come to grips with the fact that you're suffering from a life-threatening disease.

- Deciding whether or not to undergo a transplant increases the emotional turmoil.

- Sometimes the decision must be made quickly to provide the greatest likelihood of success, adding more stress to an already difficult situation.

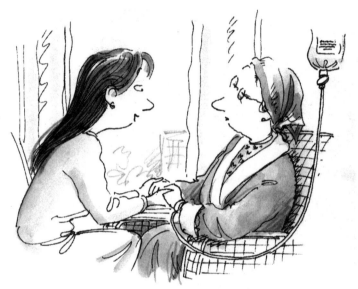

The sheer volume of information can be overwhelming. Lack of familiarity with medical jargon makes understanding doctors' explanations more difficult. It is difficult to absorb new information while still struggling with so many other details about your disease. You may ask the same question repeatedly.

It takes time to fully understand the process and it is fine to keep asking until the answer makes sense to you.

Little of the information you receive will sound like good news. What you want to hear is that the transplant will be a quick, painless, risk-free procedure. More importantly, you want assurance that it will cure you of the disease and provide you with many extra years of life. Unfortunately, no such assurances can be given. You can only be promised the chance for a future.

Fear that more unsettling news is forthcoming precludes many from asking questions. As much as you may want answers, you may opt to cope with not knowing rather than open yourself up to more disturbing information.

> Keep in mind that if something is worrying you and there is an answer, it is usually easier to live with what you know than to live with fearing the worst. That is true even if what you hear is not what you want to hear.

Getting Information

Doctors strive hard to give you a complete and honest description of the transplant experience. They want you to be fully informed about possible risks before undergoing the procedure.

In doing so, however, doctors sometimes confuse and overwhelm patients. They may assume that you are familiar with medical terms like catheters, aspirates and biopsies. Often that is not the case. As one patient put it, "doctors talk medical, patients talk human."

Don't be embarrassed to ask your doctor to repeat something or to translate it into words that you can understand. Sometimes, asking one of the nurses to explain what the doctor means will help you better understand the message.

- It helps to write down any questions you have before visiting with your doctor.

- Have a family member or friend accompany you to the visit who can help you recall important details.

- Some patients find that recording or videotaping discussions with the transplant team helps answer questions that later arise.

- Others find that keeping an ongoing file with brochures, handouts, personal notes, and resource information can be useful to refer to throughout the process.

"Your mind is going to explode with all the things you have to remember or want to ask. Write down the questions you want to ask as well as the doctor's answers to your questions. If you don't get a straight answer or don't understand the answer, ask again until it is clear."

"It's important to make sure that the doctor talks with you about the items on YOUR agenda, not just his. You need to be assertive. My 23-year-old daughter, for example, wanted to talk about infertility and options for having a child after the transplant. The doctors wanted to brush that issue aside."

Putting Things into Perspective

For many patients, the list of possible complications is frightening and overwhelming. Ask your doctor to help you put them into perspective.

- Don't assume that the risk of death or severe organ damage, for example, is as great as the risk of temporary hair loss or mouth sores. (It's not!)

- Ask what the probability is that various complications will occur. You may find it helpful to group possible complications into three categories: those that will definitely occur, those that often occur and those that rarely occur. It can help ease your worries.

Doctors sometimes forget to mention that pain relief will be provided when needed. Thus, when you hear about the numerous complications that can occur, you might assume you'll be in terrible pain. While there may be some painful complications associated with the transplant, there are a variety of effective pain medications available. (For more about pain see Chapter Thirteen, Relieving Pain.)

Setting Goals

The time spent preparing for, undergoing and recovering from a blood stem cell transplant can seem never-ending. Patients seldom make daily progress by leaps and bounds. Each day will bring a small step forward, maybe a little backsliding, or no change at all.

This slow pace of progress can be discouraging for you and your loved ones who want desperately for you to get well and put this chapter of life behind you.

Ask the doctors and nurses to help you set realistic goals, and to tell you each time progress is made, no matter how small. You may feel constantly overwhelmed by bad news. Any progress or positive news, no matter how small, can lift your spirits.

> "Progress can be so very slow. I found it was helpful to keep charts so that I could see that progress was being made. Drinking an ounce of water an hour adds up to a lot of fluid by the end of the day. Walking three feet today and increasing it by two feet each day is a lot by the end of the week."

> It helps to take one day at a time rather than worry about what will happen in five days, five weeks or five years. Focus on what you can control today when you set your goals. Prioritize what is most important for you today that you control, so you feel accomplished when you have met that goal.

Loss of Control

> "In the beginning, I was a very angry patient. I was very bitter and scared. Anger was my way of coping."

A transplant is a physically debilitating experience. You will be in a fragile state of health for several weeks following the transplant, and may feel extremely weak and helpless. Walking without assistance, focusing on a book or television show, following the thread of a conversation, or even sitting up in bed may require more energy than you have to spare.

If you are used to being in charge, taking care of yourself, or being the person upon whom others depend, you may find feeling so weak upsetting. The loss of control can bring both fear and anger. Your anger may be directed at physicians, other medical personnel or at loved ones.

It helps to remember that a loved one will be your advocate while you are too weak to fend for yourself. If you need pain relief, have questions, or need some other form of help, being able to rely on a loved one to track down the appropriate medical personnel and get the problem solved can be an immense relief.

Sometimes the best way to feel safe when you feel you do not have the energy to take charge of your needs is to give the job to a loved one you trust. This can be as simple as saying to a family member 'can you be in charge of telling the doctor I need something more for pain?'

Isolation

The special precautions taken to protect you against infection while your immune system is recovering may make you feel lonely and isolated. Most patients crave a normal environment where

- they're not the center of attention
- they can interact freely with family and friends
- they can think about something other than the disease and treatment

While you are hospitalized or staying in a facility near the hospital, rather than at home, decorate the room with things that are special to you. It can make you feel less detached from normal life.

- Keep pictures of family members on hand.
- Display cards and well wishes.
- Hang favorite pictures chosen by you on the walls, if permitted.
- Bring in your own bed clothes, books, a computer or other belongings to make your room seem homier.

> When family and friends call or visit, encourage them to talk about the world outside. Positive, upbeat anecdotes about family members and friends, descriptions of stores or museums visited, plays or movies that have seen, the latest gossip from work or school — anything that brings the outside world to you — will make you feel less isolated and cut off from normal life.

Stressful Side Effects

Some side effects of the high-dose chemotherapy and/or radiation as well as post-transplant medications and complications can be stressful.

- Temporary hair loss can change your self-image, making you self conscious or embarrassed to be seen by family and friends. Wearing a head scarf, turban, or hat may make you feel less conspicuous and can be more comfortable than a wig.

- Mouth sores, a common side effect of treatment, can make eating uncomfortable. Some of the drugs administered during treatment may temporarily alter the taste of foods. (For more on eating difficulties see Chapter Twelve, Nutrition.)

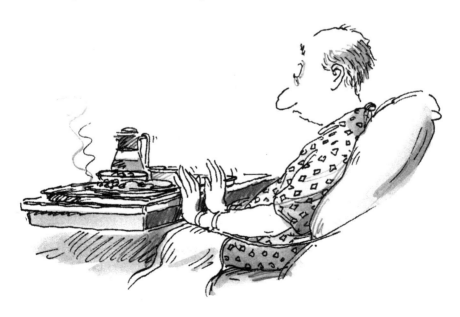

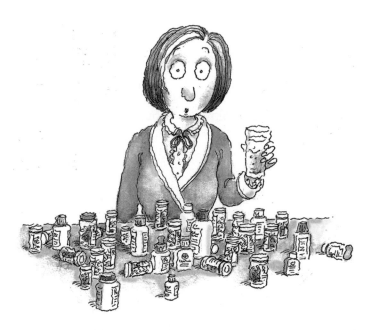

- The large quantity of medications that you will need to take each day may be overwhelming and you may have difficulty trying to force down the pills.

- The daily tests to monitor your overall physical condition, while not painful, can leave you feeling like your body is under constant assault.

In some cases, it is possible to reduce the physical discomfort associated with a procedure and thus reduce stress. Having light sedation prior to a bone marrow aspiration, for example, can make the procedure more comfortable. You should not be reluctant to ask for pre-medication or other pain relief if you are worried about discomfort.

Your family members should take an active, aggressive role in advising physicians and nurses of your discomfort and needs. Family members know your personality best and will know the extent to which you will be stoic about pain and discomfort before asking for help.

The medical team needs to know if you will request relief as soon as pain begins or only after the discomfort is really intense. The speed with which they respond to your call for help is often influenced by this important information. (For more about pain relief, see Chapter Thirteen, Relieving Pain.)

Managing Anxiety or Depression

Anxiety and distress are a normal and an expected part of the transplant experience. These are very normal reactions to a very stressful experience.

> "During my transplant I was very depressed. My dad asked a co-worker, who was five years post-transplant, to visit me and share what he had been through. He said my feelings were acceptable, that he had been depressed, too, but now he's better and working full-time. I could look at him and see that he was a normal person. That helped me more than anything."

A lot of chemicals are put into your body to cure you and relieve symptoms. These chemicals can impact your brain and feelings even while they are helping your body.

You may benefit from the services of a psychiatrist, psychologist or social worker. If your physician does not volunteer these helpful services to you, ask for them.

You may be surprised or embarrassed if you have trouble coping with anxiety on your own. This is particularly true if you have never before sought mental health services.

Needing help to cope with your emotions during treatment is normal. If you need counseling or the help of psychiatrist, it does not mean that you are falling apart, or that you will require ongoing services after recovery.

> "It's important to be honest with your own feelings. If you need help dealing with what you are about to face, seek it. This is not a sign of weakness. Sometimes, talking with someone who's been through the situation helps you separate, evaluate and move in a healthier direction."

Psychiatrists may help you manage anxiety or depression with medication. Short-term use of these drugs by transplant patients is common and should not lead to long-term drug dependency.

Insomnia

Difficulty sleeping is common among transplant recipients. Deprived of sleep, you can quickly become exhausted, unfocused and extremely irritable, making it even harder to cope with daytime stresses.

Your healthcare team may be able to provide you with medication to help you sleep. There's no need to put up with sleepless nights and the stress they produce.

> "Right before the transplant I had a lot of trouble sleeping. The whole thing was such a shock. Eventually a friend of mine, who is a pediatrician, suggested I get a prescription for sleeping pills. They really helped and they weren't addictive."

> "I had trouble sleeping when going through my transplant, and still do sometimes. I found that active relaxation helps. Rather than laying there trying to relax, I get up and do some exercises — a few leg lifts or sit ups. It helps me relax and get back to sleep."

Cognitive behavioral therapy for insomnia may also help you sleep without medication. (For more about cognitive behavioral therapy for insomnia, go to Chapter Sixteen, Late Effects in Adults and Children.)

Keeping in Touch With Friends

Throughout much of the treatment and recovery period, you may be too weak to visit with guests or even accept phone calls. Nonetheless, it's encouraging to know that family members, friends, and co-workers are concerned about your progress and hoping for your recovery.

Cards, emails, and words of encouragement from family members or friends can mean a lot when you're feeling isolated.

"My family and friends put together an album for me when I was in the hospital, and everyone contributed something. There were pictures and all sorts of silly things — it was wonderful. Another friend, who is a professional photographer, gathered everyone in the park, took their picture and blew it up. I'm talking poster-size. It included everyone — my family, my friends, my coworkers — everyone. I loved it."

Online services like CaringBridge.org are a great way to keep in touch with family and friends. CaringBridge allows you or your caregiver to create a personal web page to post daily updates about your progress for people to read. Visitors to your site can leave news about what's going on in the outside world as well as words of encouragement for you.

Sometimes people are afraid to intrude and therefore do not call or write. You can designate a close family member for people to check with before reaching out to you.

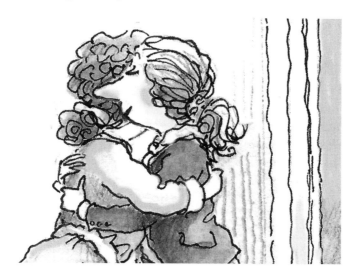

Family members, friends and co-workers sometimes have difficulty reestablishing a relationship with you after treatment. You will look different. You may have lost weight, be wearing a face mask to protect against infection, look physically drained, or have no hair. Because you will have been out of circulation for several weeks, you will not have shared as many experiences with family members or friends as usual.

> "I had one friend who was so afraid to come near me that when she would visit, she'd drive up to the front of the house, beep her horn, wave to me and then drive off. That really hurt. Others would come right into my house, put on rubber gloves, help wash and feed me — they were wonderful. They will always be my dearest and closest friends."

Friends may be unsure about how and when to re-establish a normal relationship and will look for a cue from you before making a move. You might try letting people know ahead of their visit that you appreciate them washing their hands when they arrive or what to expect when they see you. Rather than expecting them to guess what you need or will want, try letting them know if you prefer a brief visit or a walk at a certain time of day, or whatever makes it possible for you to enjoy their visit.

And Many Months Beyond

While memories of the transplant experience dim with time, it may take months before you can get through a single day without reflecting on the transplant experience. This is the natural way that our bodies and brains make sense of unfamiliar, dramatic experiences or even traumas. Innocent remarks or events totally unrelated to the transplant may stir up unpleasant memories, leaving you shaken.

> "I used to get flashbacks for about a year after my transplant. I remember walking down the aisle of a grocery store, and I'd remember something about the transplant and get a big hit of adrenaline. But that pretty much ended when I made a conscious decision to stop worrying about relapse and the transplant."

During the first year after a transplant, you may find it hard to make long-term plans or commitments.

> "In the beginning, fear of relapse definitely affected my ability to make long-term commitments. I wouldn't start

new projects or even pick out new clothes. I don't think I'll ever put it totally behind me, but I don't dwell on it anymore."

You may find it difficult to talk about your transplant, particularly with someone not intimately involved in the experience. Be kind to yourself. It will take time to get back to feeling like yourself. Your brain has been through a lot along with your body. It can take a year or more for your memory or your ability to process information to recover. This not only impacts your thinking but also your feelings. Remind yourself 'I've been through a lot and it's ok if I'm not ready to take on the whole world yet.'

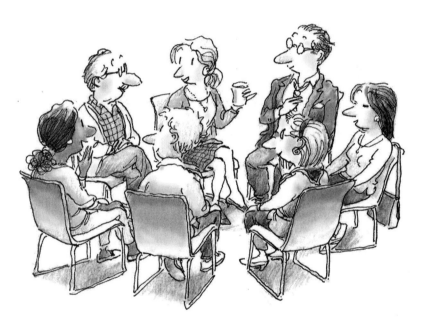

You may want an outlet to talk about the experience. Support groups are helpful for some survivors, while others prefer one-on-one discussions with counselors, other transplant survivors, a family member or a friend.

> "The support group taught me how to talk about life's most difficult problems. The people in the group share the bond of an incredibly traumatic journey, and we're not afraid to help each other."

Chapter Seven: Emotional Challenges

now Facebook groups and discussion lists on the internet
nsplant recipients and their caregivers can communicate
rs who have been through transplant. You can find links
n BMT InfoNet's website at bmtinfonet.org/emotional-challenges.

Despite the emotional upheaval a transplant causes, life after transplant can be very special. Survivors no longer take the future for granted, regardless of how promising their prognosis may be, and often enjoy each day of living more fully. As the months of survival turn into years, you will experience the added pleasure of being able once again to look forward to many more years of life.

> "Each day is special for me. When I get up in the morning, I look at the grass and trees and marvel at how beautiful everything is. For me, the transplant was like starting over again. It gave me a whole new life."

To learn more go to our website at:

bmtinfonet.org/emotional-challenges

Chapter Eight

WHEN YOUR CHILD NEEDS A TRANSPLANT

It was like a whirlwind, a dream. One day our child was a normal 15-year-old boy who would live to be 80. The next day we were staring at blackboard diagrams about transplants, and hearing doctors tell us our son might die. It wasn't real. We didn't understand. All we could do was hug each other and cry.

Lorraine, mother of 11-year transplant survivor

'Your child needs a transplant' are some of the most difficult words a parent can hear. The uncertainty, feeling of helplessness, emotional stress and fatigue associated with deciding whether or not to proceed to transplant affects the entire family.

- Young children may demonstrate rebellious or babyish behavior.

- Teens may express anger toward loved ones, engage in risky behavior or attempt to shut parents out.

- Young siblings may worry that they caused the disease or resent the extra attention their brother or sister receives.

- Stress in your marital relationship may intensify as everyone tries to cope with the difficult situation.

One thing is true: a transplant is a family affair. Acknowledging that everyone feels scared, but that everyone is working hard to make your child well can help your family pull together to face the challenges ahead. Sharing age-appropriate information with your child and siblings about the disease and treatment is important.

Through everything, remember this: thousands of children have been through a transplant and are now living normal, healthy lives.

Deciding on a Transplant

Choosing whether or not to proceed with a transplant is a difficult decision. The odds of success must be weighed against the certainty that the transplant will be a lengthy, rigorous procedure. There is often no clear-cut right choice, and you and your children can be frustrated about having to choose between several unpleasant options.

Getting easy-to-understand information prior to making a decision about a transplant is not always easy. Some transplant centers provide only oral explanations of what to expect, while others provide written materials, such as this book.

> The amount of information you receive can be overwhelming. It helps to have more than one adult present during meetings with medical personnel and to keep a journal of notes.

Sometimes parents receive conflicting information from their referring physician and the transplant team. The doctors may quote different survival rates or disagree about the timing of the transplant. Often, you are not told about all the complications associated with a transplant until you meet with the transplant team.

> "The first conference with the transplant team was the most depressing experience of my life — worse than when my daughter was diagnosed. The doctor that referred us to the transplant center never told us about the possible side effects. I was terrified. I just wanted to grab my child and run."

Don't be shy about asking questions, even if you feel it's the hundredth time the question has been asked. Bring a written list of

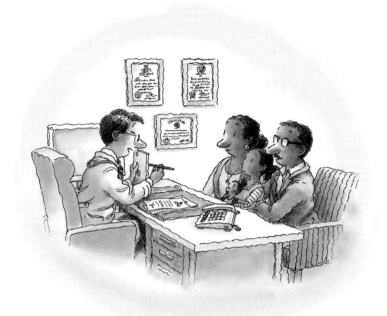

questions to your meeting with doctors and keep asking until you feel you have enough information to make a decision. It is the medical team's job to make sure all questions are answered, no matter how long or how many repetitions it takes.

Let your child ask questions as well. It is important to involve your child in the decision-making process and secure his or her cooperation and trust.

Many parents find it helpful to talk to other parents whose child went through a transplant. BMT InfoNet's Caring Connections Program can put you in contact with other parents. To access this service go to bmtinfonet.org/caring-connection or phone 888-597-7674. Keep in mind, however, that no two families' experiences will be exactly alike.

Parents, particularly if their child is under age 14, are responsible for making the final decision in most states. Nonetheless, you know it is your child who must live with the consequences and this can create internal turmoil.

> "'I knew it was a do or die situation but I kept asking myself, 'Do I really have the right to decide his life? I want to keep him with me as long as possible. Am I deciding what's best for me or for him?'"

Disagreements between parents or between parents and children about the wisdom of proceeding with a transplant are common.

> "We had just gotten our son back to the point where he seemed happy and healthy and now they were proposing a transplant. I kept thinking, 'Why take him back to ground zero? Why can't we leave him alone?' "

Listen to each other carefully, advises a transplant nurse who has witnessed many such disagreements, and respect others' concerns as much as your own.

It's a Family Affair

Once a decision has been made to proceed with a transplant, the treatment should be carefully explained to siblings. Involving siblings in discussions about your child's disease and treatment early on helps unite the family. It may also make siblings feel less resentful about the attention your sick child is receiving.

> "We decided our 12-year-old son and his brother would be told honestly about what was happening, and both would participate in decision-making as much as their age and maturity allowed. Although this placed a burden of maturity on both sons, they rose to meet it and our family drew closer, frequently drawing support from each other."

Families who involve siblings in discussions about the child's care and treatment often have fewer problems later on with sibling jealousy or anger. Be completely honest with both your sick child and his or her siblings from the start so there are no surprises down the road and no feelings that they've been lied to, say psychologists who work with transplant patients.

Your Child's Donor

If a sibling is to be the bone marrow or stem cell donor, it's important that his or her questions are answered as well. It's easy to forget that the donor is a patient too with questions and worries. Explaining and demonstrating the medical procedure to the donor, and assuring the child that a parent or loved one will be there with him or her can help ease the donor's fears.

While it may be tempting to encourage the sibling donor by saying how important his or her role will be in saving your sick child's life, that puts a lot of pressure and responsibility on a child and may create problems later if the transplant does not succeed.

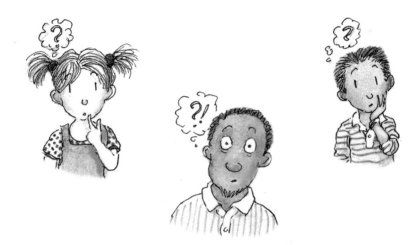

Questions Children Ask

Children's questions and concerns about the transplant vary depending on their age. Younger children focus on immediate problems and ask questions such as:

- How much it will hurt?
- Will I be separated from my parents?
- When can I return to school?
- When will my hair will grow back?
- Will I vomit a lot?
- Will I have chemotherapy again?

After acquiring a basic understanding of the procedure, younger children tend to rely on their parents to decide what's best.

Teens, on the other hand, take a much more active role in the decision-making process and, by law, must give their consent to the procedure in most states.

Teens may be concerned with:

- self-image, such as hair loss
- fitting in with peers after transplant
- infertility and sexuality

The possibility of infertility post-transplant can be distressing for an adolescent. Sexual identity and activity are important to teens. Many don't understand the distinction between being fertile and being sexually active.

It helps to tell them that many adults are infertile, yet lead a normal sex life. It's also important to help them distinguish between childbearing and child rearing.

Introducing the Hospital and Equipment

Before undergoing a transplant, children should be introduced to the:

- hospital
- transplant team
- equipment that will be used, such as catheters and IV poles

They should be given simple, clear explanations about what these devices do, why they are needed, and what it will feel like when they are used.

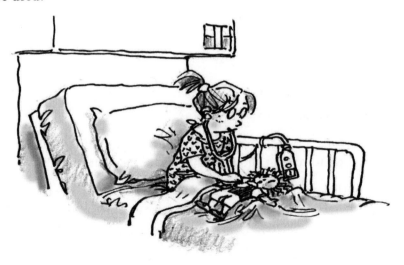

Allowing younger children to handle the hospital equipment and try out the procedures on dolls before they enter the hospital often helps them get comfortable with the equipment and allows them to ask questions.

Bringing siblings to the hospital and showing them where their brother or sister will spend the next several weeks is also a good idea if the transplant center allows this. They will feel less left out and will have a better sense of where their sibling will be and what will be done.

Coping With Anxiety

Once preparations for the transplant have been finalized, families can feel uneasy. Everyone will be anxious, and you may agonize over the wisdom of proceeding with this treatment.

> "You have to learn to have confidence in your ability to make decisions, and believe you made the best choice under the circumstance. Don't panic about what may happen, and don't fret about what has happened. It can't be changed. Just take one day at a time."

For most children, the transplant will be the hardest challenge they've ever faced.

- Younger children may fear that they are to blame for the disease and treatment. They may think they were somehow bad and are now being punished.

- Young siblings may also fear that they caused the problem. They may recall getting angry with the sick child and saying or thinking 'I wish you'd get sick or die' and now it is coming to pass.

> It's important that children of all ages be encouraged to discuss their feelings openly so their concerns can be addressed. Find out what your child is thinking. Don't assume that if he or she doesn't talk about the illness or transplant there's no problem.

Some children express their anxieties through behavioral changes. Behavioral changes to look for include:

- belligerence
- depression
- poor performance in school
- regression to behavior typical of younger children

> Let your children know that you understand they're unhappy, frightened and confused, and that you are unhappy too. Assure them that everyone will work hard to make your child well again.

Sometimes children will more openly discuss their feelings with someone other than their parents. This is particularly true of pre-teens and adolescents who are fearful of hurting their parents' feelings or causing them distress. Adolescents who are coping with typical teen desires for independence may be especially reluctant to let down their guard in the presence of parents.

It's important to allow children to discuss their feelings with whomever they feel most comfortable. You can seek the help of nurses, psychologists or other counselors to encourage your child to talk about his or her concerns.

Life During Transplant

Although a transplant is anything but routine, it is important to maintain as much of your child's normal home routine as possible.

- Bring favorite clothes, pictures, and toys to the hospital to maintain a sense of normalcy.
- Arrange for calls, letters and/or visits from your child's classmates, favorite teacher, church members, or your hometown doctor with whom your child feels comfortable.
- Some families make videos of family and friends that their child can view while in the hospital.

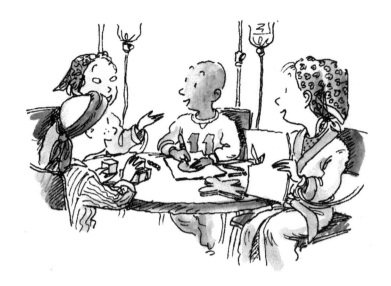

- Facetime and Zoom allow children to interact with family and friends remotely and can be very uplifting.

Boredom in the hospital can be a big issue for children. Planning diversions and activities for teens is especially important.

> "My son, who was 15 years old, was transplanted at a children's hospital. Although they had lots of activities planned, they were usually geared toward younger kids, not teens."

Loss of Control

Despite everyone's best efforts, the hospitalization will be a very stressful time for you and your child. Your child will be inundated with tests, medications and daily medical procedures.

Children of all ages, and teens in particular, feel overwhelmed by all the rules and bosses and can become angry over the loss of personal control. This can manifest itself in a variety of ways.

- Some children refuse to eat or play.
- Others may become depressed, listless or exhibit regressive or babyish behavior. They may be incapable of performing tasks they were previously able to do on their own.

Parents usually bear the brunt of the behavioral changes.

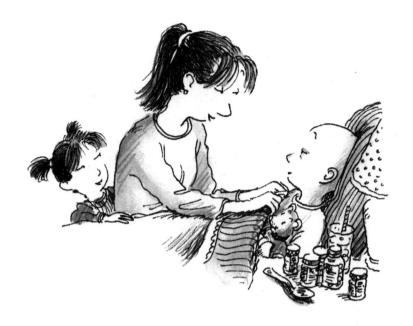

> Children spend a whole lot of time and energy growing up, seizing control over their life, and becoming more independent. When they undergo a transplant, they lose that independence and control, and that can make them angry or depressed.

Children don't feel the same urgency about routine medical procedures as parents do. It's important to talk with children and let them know that you know it's hard, and that feeling angry is normal and okay.

> "I never said to my son, 'don't cry'. I encouraged him to talk about what was bothering him and to let it all out. If he really rebelled against doing something like mouth care, I wouldn't insist it be done that moment. We'd talk about it and usually it would get done without a fight five minutes later. Sometimes I'd suggest we do it a few minutes before the nurse came in so that he could feel like it was his decision and not her order that made it happen. He liked that feeling of control."

> Children are as concerned about protecting their bodies and having control over their personal life as adults. Don't violate their bodies without asking permission. Give them the opportunity to say no or to make choices regarding their care or daily activities whenever it's possible for you to honor their decision.

Setting up and sticking to a daily routine in the hospital is important for children. Ideally, the routine should include some safe time for the child each day during which no unpleasant tests, medications, or staff interventions occur.

Preparing for Medical Procedures

Preparing children for each new medication or medical procedure is very important.

- Explain what will be done.
- Show or explain what the equipment will look like.
- Explain how they will feel during the procedure.

Children should be told about the medication or procedure far enough in advance to allow them to work through questions, but not so far in advance that they have time to brood about it.

It helps to allow children to rehearse medical procedures in advance, or to practice the procedure on dolls or adults. Break the procedure into small steps, moving on to the next step only after the child's anxiety about the first step has been relieved.

Advance explanation is even required before the administration of drugs designed to ease pain or sedate the child.

> "The first time my child was given Demerol® he became almost violent. He wasn't prepared for the fact that he'd feel groggy and it frightened him. After that, I always made sure he knew in advance how the drugs would make him feel."

You are an important advocate for your child, particularly when it comes to securing pain relief or minimizing the discomfort associated with medical procedures. Some centers, for example, give sedatives or other pain control medications to children in advance of a bone marrow aspirate (a medical procedure that can be very uncomfortable) while others do not. Don't hesitate to ask for pain medication if your child has difficulty with a procedure.

Challenges for Parents

The time in the hospital is difficult for parents. It's hard to watch your child undergo difficult medical procedures, particularly when you have so little control over his or her care.

> "They kept saying that being there for my child was important but it never felt like I was doing enough."

It is important to pace yourself during this time so that you don't become exhausted or ill. Taking a few minutes off while social workers or visitors spend time with your child can be helpful. Some parents find that spending the night away from the hospital enables them to get a good night's rest and better cope with the next day's stresses. For other parents, remaining with their child overnight is less stressful.

> "My mother and sister would sometimes stay with my son while I went to a nearby mall or got my hair done. Just getting outside, even for a few minutes, made a tremendous difference."

> "At first it was hard for me to leave my child each night, and I tried to get the hospital to change their policy. But it became a haven for me — I could take a hot bath, watch television, sleep and have some time to myself."

Children are very perceptive about their parents' feelings and can be frightened when they detect sadness or stress in their parents. Some children may feel guilty, thinking they caused their parents' sadness, and a desire to protect their parents can be a stumbling block to speaking frankly about their own concerns. Acknowledging that the hospitalization is scary for everyone, and that you will work through the experience together is important.

> "Every day my son would say, 'I love you. Thank you for being here with me. It makes it easier when I'm not feeling good.' He knew it was just as hard for me as it was for him."

Siblings' Care

Often siblings must be left in the care of friends or relatives while their brother or sister is undergoing a transplant. This may involve removing them from their home and normal routines. Young children may view this separation from their parents as a punishment.

It is important that siblings know that you don't want to be away from them, that the separation will be temporary and why it's not possible for them to be with you.

Setting up a plan of routine contact between the parents and siblings will ease the feeling that they are being ignored or that they aren't loved as much as the sick child.

> "Every day I would call my daughter and send her a note. When I wrote, I would tell her what was happening with her brother, but when I called, I made sure we talked about her."

Marital Stress

It is not unusual for problems that previously existed in a marriage to be heightened during this time. Plans for a separation or divorce may get put on hold as a result of the transplant, with tensions between marital partners increasing. Substance abuse problems may worsen as a result of the added stress.

Don't be embarrassed to seek help for these problems — you won't be the first. In general, it's best to make as few changes as possible in the home routine and keep lines of communication open during this difficult time.

Even if you feel you have a good relationship you can still experience severe marital tensions. One parent — usually the mother — remains at the hospital with the child, while the spouse spends most of his time at home, continuing to work, taking care of the home and caring for the other children. Both may be thrust into roles they normally don't assume.

The caregiver at the hospital must deal with complicated medical issues, a child who is physically and emotionally exhausted, and his or her own exhaustion and emotions. This person gets little or no break from the stress.

The spouse at home may assume more child care and household responsibilities, and must deal with his own fears as well as the emotional needs of his other children. He may feel left out or poorly informed about the day-to-day medical aspects of what's happening with the sick child.

Both are under stress and need each other's support. However, both are often too exhausted or upset to understand how the other spouse feels and what he or she needs. As one mother put it, "Stress like this will either make a marriage stronger or pull it apart."

> "I was at the hospital 24-hours-a-day. My husband was able to re-enter the world when he became overwhelmed, go to the office and pretend to live a normal life. When we came home, he wanted things to return to normal, but I was just starting to process what we had been through. I was coping with the anger and fear I couldn't focus on in the hospital. I was extremely angry that he couldn't see things the way I did. One night I felt like our marriage was over. I told him he didn't understand where I'd been. He said, 'I've been there, too.' We went to therapy together and were able to address a lot of issues."

> "I was a raving lunatic and my husband didn't understand why. I was dead tired and would have liked for him to pick up the slack. He couldn't do it. He was devastated when our child got sick — he'd never had to handle a catastrophe like this before. Sometimes, I just needed a big hug from him but he wasn't capable of it. I got mad and snippy with him when he wouldn't do little things like take out the garbage without being asked. I started to resent him. I finally realized that if you have bad feelings, you have to talk about it — even if your husband isn't a talker. It takes work to keep a marriage together under these circumstances — it's not a piece of cake."

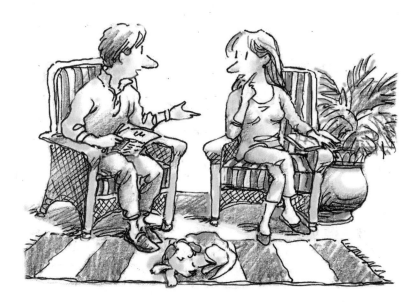

"It's important to respect each other's differences. I think men and women handle crises in different ways. My husband and I handled our fears differently — one way is not necessarily better than the other."

Going Home

Going home — the day that everyone waits for — can be a bittersweet experience. Although the hospitalization has ended, the recovery period is far from over.

Medications must be administered several times daily, central lines must be cleaned, and several visits per week must be made to the outpatient clinic to monitor progress.

You and your spouse will be on pins and needles watching for signs of infection or other complications.

"You think you'll get to go home and lead a normal life but it's not like that. Living at home with a child who has a weak immune system is scary. We were constantly worrying that my husband would bring home germs from work, and we carried disinfectant everywhere."

It is common for problems to develop that require the child to be readmitted to the hospital for a short time. This can be alarming for parents and children alike.

> "You never know what will come up. Since we've come home, we've had many trips to the hospital. There's still a lot of home care for our daughter, even now. She still has the central line, the feeding tube, and lots of medications to take. Every time something goes wrong I feel guilty, thinking that something I did made my child worse. Wrong thoughts, I know, but we're only human."

Sometimes, behavioral problems surface after transplant. Parents are set up to be in an awkward position. While in the hospital, the child may get lots of cards, gifts, balloons and attention, and may expect it to continue when he or she returns home.

Frequently, friends and extended family fail to understand that the trauma continues long after a child returns home.

> "They think that once you walk out the door of the hospital, everything is behind you, and you should pick up life where you left off. It just doesn't work that way."

> "It would really drive me crazy when people would say, 'You must feel so lucky' or 'You must be so grateful' when I was feeling anything but lucky. While I was grateful to have witnessed a miracle, I was still really angry that our family had to go through all this."

The reunion of the siblings with the parent who spent time at the hospital is not always a smooth one.

> "At first my three-year-old refused to talk to me. My daughter was left in my husband's care at home during my son's transplant. She talked with my husband and treated him like her parent, but closed up to me. That hurt a lot. We found a therapist who helped us understand her fears and resentments, and work through them."

Siblings can become jealous about the extra attention the transplant survivor receives after returning home. They may express a desire to be sick so their mother will pay more attention to them. They can resent the fact that different rules apply to them than to the transplant child.

Some parents find that involving siblings in the routine caregiving can make them feel needed and important. Setting aside time for the parent and sibling to do something special together also helps.

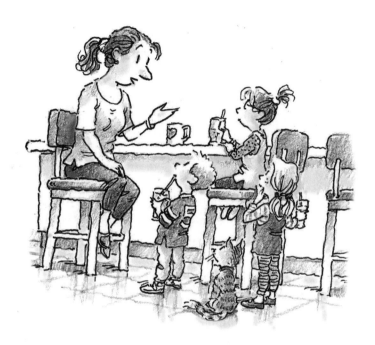

"My four-year-old daughter was not pleased when my son came home from the hospital. There was a lot of whining, crying and naughtiness like biting. She directed her anger at me, not my son. I tried to find special things for her — like special times for her to be with her parents or special treats when we'd take my son to the clinic. That seemed to help."

"My five-year-old cried a lot. She kept asking, 'Why is my sister always sick? Why does she get extra attention?' I told her that I loved them equally, and I talked with her about what it was like when she was a little baby like her sister. I told her mommy was with her the whole time and paid lots of attention to her. I said, 'It's okay to be angry, but it's not your sister's fault — don't be angry with her.' I feel like I missed a good bit of my five-year-old because I was so preoccupied with the baby and her problems from birth. Now I try to make up the difference in healthy ways."

Getting Back to Normal

Getting back to normal will be a slow process. For many months after the transplant, both the transplant recipient and siblings may become anxious over symptoms of a common cold or other minor discomforts.

"I went to my son's room one night when I heard him sniffling. 'This feels so familiar,' he said. 'I always used to get sick at night and you'd have to take me to the hospital.' When I assured him that he would be okay, he said, 'That sounds familiar, too.'"

"Our daughter was afraid to get sick after her brother's transplant. When she got the flu last week it was the first time that she was the sick one rather than her brother. He hovered over her, rubbed her back, and brought her something to drink, trying to soothe her. They were both very concerned."

Don't assume siblings' complaints of illness are a deliberate ploy to get attention, advises a psychologist. Children often mimic symptoms of the illness unconsciously and truly believe they are ill.

> Don't ignore or trivialize a sibling's complaints of illness. Show them you are as concerned about their well-being as you are about the child who had a transplant. Call the doctor even if you think it is something minor. It can help put their mind at ease.

Certain events that parents view as milestones can be very traumatic for your child. A two-year-old, for example, became very upset when his central line was removed.

> "We thought he'd be happy to get rid of it. Instead, he became very upset — it was like part of his body was being removed."

Returning to school is a milestone that children are often encouraged to look forward to, but it, too, can be a tremendous letdown.

- They may find their classmates are not anxiously awaiting their return.
- Their friends may have moved on to new interests and activities without them.
- Some children may be afraid to associate with a child who has been sick and now looks different.

It helps to prepare classmates in advance for the child's return. A nurse, doctor or social worker can visit the school, explain what has happened to the child, and answer questions.

The Leukemia & Lymphoma Society offers the Trish Greene Back to School Program to help children and teachers with a child's transition back to school. Call 800-955-4572 for more details.

Despite the difficulties, the transplant experience often brings families closer together:

> "My children still squabble a lot, but they're very concerned and protective of each other as well. It was rough while we went through it, but the good times have come now. My son made it, he's healthy, and we all appreciate what it means to be alive."

To learn more go to our website at:
bmtinfonet.org/talking-children-about-transplants

Chapter Nine
PREPARATIVE/ CONDITIONING REGIMEN

The doctor spent thirty minutes telling me all the things that could go wrong. Suddenly I could hear no more. 'Stop,' I said emphatically. 'I know you have to give me all the statistics, but I am not a statistic. My name is Harvey and I have an attitude problem. I refuse to die. Now, I believe that I can make it, do you?'

Harvey, three-year transplant survivor

The preparative regimen (also called the conditioning regimen) is the high-dose chemotherapy and/or radiation you will receive in the days prior to your transplant.

The preparative regimen has two objectives:

- to destroy your disease

- to suppress your immune system so that your donor's blood stem cells can engraft and begin producing healthy blood cells.

Drugs used in the preparative regimen are sometimes the same as those used in standard chemotherapy to treat the disease. The dosages, however, are much higher and more effective in killing the disease.

High-Dose Chemotherapy

Most preparative regimens include high-dose chemotherapy. The chemotherapy drugs are usually administered intravenously over a one-to-six day period through a catheter that is placed in a large vein near your chest. If the chemotherapy drug busulfan is part of the preparative regimen, it may be given to you intravenously or as a pill.

Total Body Irradiation (TBI)

Some preparative regimens include total body irradiation. TBI is used most often in transplants for patients with leukemia, lymphoma, and severe aplastic anemia.

Total body irradiation is typically administered to patients in one or more sessions over a one-to-seven day period. When TBI is given over several days, it is called fractionated TBI. If it is broken up into several lower-dosage sessions in a single day it is called hyperfractionated TBI.

You will not actually see or feel the radiation, but you may still find TBI therapy an unnerving experience.

- You will sit or lie still, sometimes in an awkward position, for 10 to 45 minutes while the radiation is being administered. This can be difficult, particularly if you are nauseated.

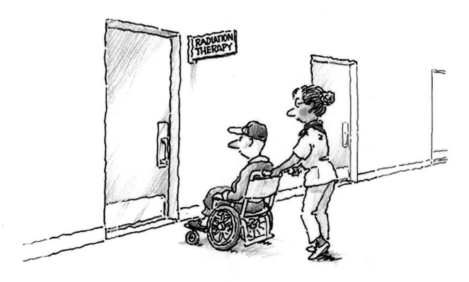

- Some transplant centers use special stands or boxes to help you remain immobile during TBI. These can be confining and make you feel anxious.

- Pre-medication with sedatives can help reduce anxiety.

- Children are usually sedated before TBI sessions to minimize their movement and very young children may even be anesthetized.

It helps to visit the radiation center before TBI therapy begins in order to familiarize yourself with the equipment and to get your questions answered. Most centers provide patients with a simulation of TBI therapy so they know, in advance, what to expect, and so that the health care team can make sure that dosages and equipment measurements are correct.

Reduced Intensity (Nonmyeloablative) Transplants

If you are having a reduced intensity or nonmyeloablative transplant, you will receive lower dosages of chemotherapy than those given to standard transplant patients. Thus, the side effects may not be as severe.

There are many different types of reduced intensity transplants. Ask your doctor to outline the potential side effects associated with the specific treatment you are about to receive.

Common Side Effects

High-dose chemotherapy and TBI are toxic to normal tissues and organs as well as diseased cells. Typical side effects include:

- nausea
- vomiting
- diarrhea
- mouth sores
- temporary hair loss

These side effects almost always occur to varying degrees regardless of which preparative regimen is used. Severe or long-term damage to organs and tissues occurs less frequently.

> It is normal to be frightened and overwhelmed by the list of possible side effects associated with the preparative regimen. Keep in mind that most side effects are temporary and completely reversible, and that severe or long-term organ damage is the exception rather than the rule.

As you read the following sections, keep in mind that the degree to which people experience side effects is different, and no one experiences all possible side effects.

Nausea, Vomiting and Diarrhea

Nausea and vomiting are common following all preparative regimens, but can be controlled with medications. Drugs called antiemetics are used to treat nausea.

Antiemetics can cause additional side effects such as

- anxiety
- drowsiness
- restlessness
- muscle tightness
- uncontrolled eye movement
- shakiness

These drug reactions can be frightening but are usually less serious than they appear. Lowering the dosage of the antiemetic or administering an antihistamine usually reduces or eliminates the problem.

Diarrhea following the preparative regimen is also common. Antidiarrheal drugs such as Lomotil® can sedate the nerves in the gastrointestinal area, slowing down muscle contractions and the diarrhea.

Mouth and Throat

High-dose chemotherapy and radiation target rapidly dividing cells like cancer cells. However, some normal cells also divide rapidly, such as those that line the mouth, throat and gut. These cells can be temporarily damaged by high-dose chemotherapy or TBI.

Mouth sores (mucositis) and throat sores (stomatitis) typically appear four-to-eight days following the preparative regimen.

- Topical anesthetics such as Dyclone®, or narcotics given intravenously such as morphine, are used to relieve this discomfort.

- Frequent brushing of the teeth and gums with a soft brush or sponge, and rinsing with a saline solution helps prevent mouth infections.

- A drug called palifermin (Kepivance®) may lessen the severity and duration of mucositis.

- There are rinses that can help reduce the discomfort caused by mouth sores.

Mucositis often makes eating difficult or impossible. You may be fed intravenously until the discomfort subsides. Intravenous feeding is also used if your stomach is unable to absorb sufficient nutrients as a result of temporary irritation caused by the preparative regimen. Antacid medication may be given to counteract stomach irritation.

Hair

Temporary hair loss (alopecia) usually occurs following the preparative regimen. Hair loss changes your appearance and, for some, can be very distressing.

- Scarves, hats or wigs can be used until the hair grows back.

- You may prefer to shave your head or cut your hair very short before hair loss begins.

- Hair normally grows back within three-to-six months following the transplant.

- Sometimes the amount of curl or thickness of the new hair will differ from your hair pre-transplant.

- In rare cases, hair loss may be permanent.

Skin

Skin rash is common following preparative regimens that include TBI, busulfan, etoposide, carmustine or thiotepa. At some centers, showers are recommended one and six hours after infusion of thiotepa to reduce the likelihood of developing a rash.

Less often, hyperpigmentation– dark spots on the skin – occurs. Hyperpigmentation is most common in patients with a darker skin tone, and is most obvious in skin creases and on fingernails and toenails. The spots usually fade in one-to-three months.

Eyes

Premature cataracts occur in approximately 20 percent of patients who undergo fractionated TBI. Cataracts may also occur following treatment with high-dose busulfan. Cataracts can be surgically removed, usually in an outpatient setting.

Bladder Irritation (hemorrhagic cystitis)

Bladder irritation, which can cause bloody or painful urination, sometimes occurs following the preparative regimen, particularly those that include cyclophosphamide or ifosfamide. Strategies to prevent or treat the problem include:

- increasing the rate of intravenous fluids
- using a catheter to irrigate the bladder
- giving a drug called MESNA®

Liver

Temporary liver damage can occur following high-dose chemotherapy and/or TBI. It is usually both mild and completely reversible.

Liver blood test abnormalities occur in approximately 50 percent of patients following the preparative regimen, but only a small fraction will develop actual liver damage. You may experience

- jaundice (yellowing of the skin)
- significant weight gain due to fluid retention

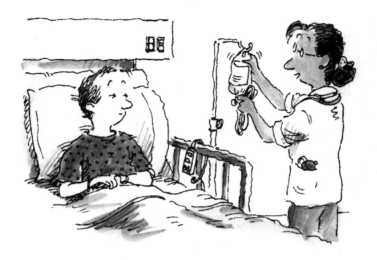

- abnormal blood levels of liver enzymes and bilirubin (a pigment produced during the break up of red blood cells)

Resting the liver and avoiding medications that aggravate the condition are the usual treatments until the liver heals itself.

Sinusoidal obstruction syndrome (SOS), previously known as veno-occlusive disease (VOD), is a potentially serious liver problem caused by high-dose chemotherapy and/or TBI.

- The blood vessels that carry blood through the liver become swollen and blocked.
- Without a supply of blood, the liver cannot remove toxins, drugs and other waste products from the bloodstream.
- Fluids build up in the liver causing swelling and tenderness.
- The kidneys may retain excess water and salt, causing swelling in the legs, arms and abdomen.

In severe cases, excess fluid in the abdominal cavity puts pressure on the lungs making it difficult to breathe. Toxins that are not processed out of the blood by the liver may affect how the brain functions and confusion may result (although confusion is a symptom of other, less serious problems as well).

A drug called defibrotide is now available to help treat this complication.

Lungs and Heart

Breathing irregularities can occur following the preparative regimen. Some patients develop pneumonia during the first four weeks after transplant. In most cases, injury to the lungs is mild and temporary but some patients do experience long-term breathing problems.

Mild, temporary heartbeat irregularities (arrhythmia) or rapid heartbeat (tachycardia) can occur following the preparative regimen, particularly those that include cyclophosphamide or carmustine. Severe heart problems are rare.

Changes in Thinking

Confusion or altered thinking is an occasional, temporary side effect of the preparative regimen, or of drugs used to control other side effects. Confusion and altered thinking can be frightening both to you and your loved ones who observe it. These problems are usually temporary and reversible, and can be managed by changing the dosage or type of drug.

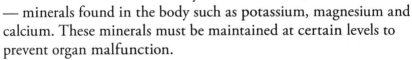

Muscle Spasms and Cramping

Muscle spasms are common after transplant. High-dose chemotherapy can cause imbalance in electrolytes — minerals found in the body such as potassium, magnesium and calcium. These minerals must be maintained at certain levels to prevent organ malfunction.

Muscle spasms can often be resolved by taking potassium, calcium, magnesium or phosphate supplements orally. Ask your doctor to prescribe the supplement, since not all sources of these minerals are absorbed equally well by the body. If there is no electrolyte imbalance, vitamin E or quinine (like the amount found in tonic water) sometimes helps.

Reproductive Organs

Most men can bank their sperm before transplant. Sperm banking may be an option even if you had prior chemotherapy. Although you may not think you want children later on, sperm banking is worth considering in case you change your mind.

> High-dose chemotherapy and radiation cause most, but not all, patients to be infertile after transplant. If you are having a reduced intensity transplant, you may not be infertile after transplant.
>
> Fortunately, there are steps you can take if you wish to have children after transplant.

For women, it may be possible to collect eggs prior to transplant, fertilize them with sperm to create embryos and then freeze the embryos for later use. It is also possible to freeze unfertilized eggs, although the success rate with unfertilized eggs is less than that with fertilized eggs. Both procedures require several weeks and may not be an option for you if you need to proceed quickly to transplant.

Another experimental option for women is freezing ovarian tissue. Ovarian tissue is removed during a short, outpatient surgical procedure and then frozen. The tissue can later be implanted into a woman's ovary where it may produce eggs.

(For information about other options to create a family after transplant go to Chapter Eighteen, Family Planning.)

Numbness and Tingling

You may experience numbness and tingling in your hands and feet due to nerve damage caused by the preparative regimen or prior chemotherapy. Usually the damage is permanent. However, in a few patients there has been slow regrowth of nerve tissue that eventually reduces numbness and tingling.

Pediatric Issues

Mild to moderate learning disabilities and memory problems may occur, particularly in children, especially if the preparative regimen includes TBI.

Young children often experience delayed growth as well. Hormone therapy may be recommended to promote growth. After transplant, children should be followed by a pediatrician with specific knowledge of growth problems.

Certain chemotherapy drugs called anthracyclines (doxorubicin, daunorubicin and mitoxantrone) and radiation can increase the risk of heart problems in pediatric transplant survivors. Although the risk is small, the problem may occur decades after treatment so patients should be monitored for heart problems long-term.

Children transplanted before the age of five may also experience significant dental problems such as loose teeth, tooth loss, and dry mouth and may be unable to wear braces. It is important that they be followed by a dentist who is experienced in treating children who had high-dose chemotherapy and/or total body irradiation.

Putting Risks in Perspective

Anxiety about the possible side effects of the preparative regimen is normal. It helps to put the risk of developing each side effect into perspective, and to remember that most are temporary and completely reversible. Counselors and psychiatrists are available at most transplant centers to help you cope with your anxiety.

> "Be prepared for complications. Very few things will happen just as described. There are many possible complications. No one gets all of them, but most get some of them. Learn to separate those that are serious, but reversible, from those that are truly life-threatening."

To learn more go to our website at:

bmtinfonet.org/preparative-regimen

Chapter Ten
GRAFT-VERSUS-HOST DISEASE

It's been a little over two years since Jon's transplant. The journey has not been easy but we survived. For now, he has gotten through his GVHD pretty well but it took a long while. His bones get sore and he has sinus difficulty, but not everything is bad. He played baseball this summer, rode his bike and skateboard, and just got home from playing floor hockey. Although not perfect, things sure are great now.

Jocelyn, mother of six-year transplant survivor

Graft-versus-host disease (GVHD) is a common complication following an allogeneic transplant.

GVHD occurs when the donor's immune system (the graft) perceives the patient's organs and tissues (the host) as unfamiliar cells that should be destroyed. The donor cells that trigger this reaction are a type of white blood cell called T-cells.

Most cases of GVHD are mild or moderate and resolve over time. However, GVHD can also be more severe and, in some cases, life-threatening.

Patients who develop GVHD usually do so during the first year after transplant. However, GVHD can also occur months or years later.

There are two types of GVHD:
- acute GVHD
- chronic GVHD

A patient may develop one, both or neither. Each type has a different effect on organs and tissues.

Although acute and chronic GVHD usually occur during different time periods after transplant, it is possible for a patient to have both at the same time.

Acute GVHD

Acute GVHD typically occurs during the first three months after transplant, although it can also occur later.

The risk of developing acute GVHD is highest in patients who were transplanted with a mismatched or unrelated donor.

Other factors that may increase the risk of developing acute GVHD include:

- total body irradiation as part of the conditioning regimen
- a female donor for a male patient
- the type of drugs used to prevent acute GVHD

Preventing Acute GVHD

To reduce the risk of developing acute GVHD, patients are usually given medications starting a day or two before transplant such as:

- cyclosporine and methotrexate
- tacrolimus and methotrexate
- cyclosporine and mycophenolate mofetil
- tacrolimus and sirolimus
- antithymocyte globulin

These drugs suppress your immune system, making it more difficult for the donor's cells to attack your organs and tissues. You may need to continue taking these drugs for several months after transplant.

Your doctor may give you additional drugs after transplant, such as cyclophosphamide, to further reduce the risk of developing acute GVHD.

At some transplant centers, the T-cells that can cause graft-versus-host disease are removed from the donor's cells prior to transplant. This procedure is called T-cell depletion.

Although T-cell depletion reduces the risk of developing GVHD, it can increase the risk of relapse or infection in some patients. Researchers are exploring whether removing a subset of T-cells from the donor's cells will protect patients against GVHD without increasing the risk of relapse and infection.

Symptoms of Acute GVHD

In most patients, acute GVHD first affects the skin causing:

- a mild or faint rash on the back, shoulders, ears or neck
- a rash on the palms of the hands or soles of the feet

The rash may resemble a sunburn with peeling or blistering, or it may look like a heat rash, and may eventually spread.

Acute GVHD can also affect the gastrointestinal tract causing:

- abdominal pain
- watery or bloody diarrhea
- persistent nausea and/or vomiting
- loss of appetite or feeling full after eating only a little

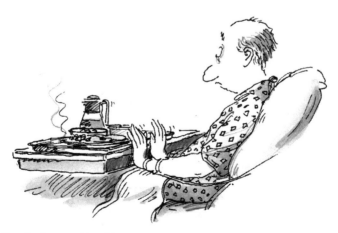

If acute GVHD affects the liver, it can cause:

- elevated liver enzyme levels
- jaundice (yellowing of skin and eyes)
- dark urine

Treatment for Acute GVHD

If you develop acute GVHD, drugs such as prednisone or methylprednisolone may help control the disease. If your GVHD does not respond to these drugs, your doctor may try other agents or treatments such as:

- ruxolitinib
- antithymocyte globulin
- sirolimus
- mycophenolate mofetil
- extracorporeal photopheresis

> Extracorporeal photopheresis is a procedure that removes some white blood cells from the patient, mixes them with a drug called psoralen, and exposes them to ultraviolet light. The cells are then reinfused into the patient.

Your doctor will begin tapering down the dosage of the drugs once it appears your acute GVHD is under control. It's possible, however, for acute GVHD to return or get worse during the tapering process. You may need to continue your GVHD medications for a longer period of time until the disease is no longer active.

Your doctor may also recommend that you enroll in a clinical trial that is testing a new therapy for GVHD. To find a GVHD clinical trial appropriate for you contact the Jason Carter Clinical Trials Program at jasoncarterclinicaltrialsprogram.org or phone 888-814-8610. You can also go to clinicaltrials.gov.

Chronic GVHD

Chronic GVHD is different than acute GVHD. It usually develops later than acute GVHD and can affect more organs and tissues.

Chronic GVHD occurs most often in patients who:

- previously had acute GVHD
- are older
- had an unrelated donor or a donor who was not a perfect match
- were transplanted with stem cells collected from the blood stream (peripheral blood stem cells), rather than bone marrow or cord blood
- are a male and received cells from a female donor
- received cells from a female donor who previously bore children

Most cases of chronic GVHD are mild or moderate. However, 10-15 percent of patients develop symptoms that are more severe.

Treatment for Chronic GVHD

How your doctor manages your chronic GVHD depends on which organs and tissues are affected, the severity of the symptoms, and impact GVHD is having on your daily life.

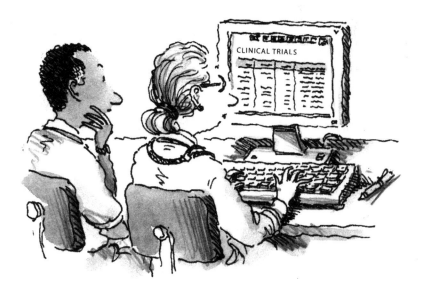

If chronic GVHD is affecting only one or two organs or tissues, your doctor may choose a localized therapy, like an ointment, to manage the disease.

If chronic GVHD is affecting many different parts of your body, or if the symptoms are severe, your doctor may treat it with drugs that suppress your immune system such as:

- prednisone
- prednisone with cyclosporine
- prednisone with tacrolimus

If your chronic GVHD does not respond well to these treatments, your doctor may try other drugs or treatments such as:

- ibrutinib
- methotrexate
- mycophenolate mofetil
- sirolimus
- extracorporeal photopheresis
- low dose interleukin-2
- ruxolitinib

Patients with chronic GVHD typically require treatment for up to three-to-five years. Approximately 15 percent of patients require treatment for a longer time period. In rare cases, some patients need life-long immunosuppressive drugs.

How Chronic GVHD Affects Skin, Nails, Hair and Sweat Glands

Chronic GVHD most often affects the skin. Symptoms may include:

- a dry, itchy rash
- a burning sensation when exposed to sun or heat
- a tightening or pulling sensation

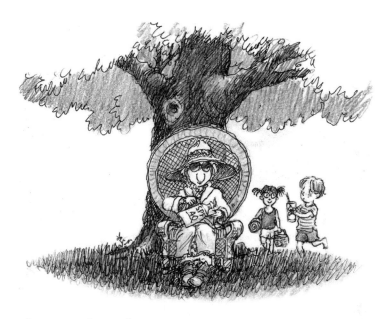

- a change in skin color
- thickening of the skin that may restrict joint movement
- taut skin
- thinning of the skin, easy skin tearing

GVHD may also cause:

- brittle or splitting fingernails and toenails
- hair loss or thinning hair
- changes in hair color or texture
- joint stiffness
- contractures (shortening or hardening of muscles and connective tissues)
- difficulty opening the mouth fully due to taut skin around the mouth
- an inability to sweat or handle heat for long periods of time, due to damaged sweat glands
- difficulty breathing, due to tight skin on the chest

- feeling full quickly because skin on the abdomen is taut
- tightening of tissue under the skin (the fascia) which can look like cellulite

Corticosteroids or tacrolimus ointment applied directly on the skin may relieve some of these symptoms. If tight skin is restricting joint movement, physical therapy may help.

If skin GVHD is causing joint stiffness or contractures, your doctor may recommend deep tissue massage and/or stretching exercises to improve your range of motion.

Extracorporeal photopheresis is another possible treatment for skin GVHD.

Your Mouth and Chronic GVHD

Chronic GVHD often affects the mouth and salivary glands. Symptoms may include:

- redness and lacey white patches in the mouth, often on the tongue or inner cheeks
- painful sores anywhere in the mouth
- sensitivity to spicy, acidic or crunchy foods, carbonated beverages and mint flavored toothpaste
- a very dry mouth, due to loss of saliva
- changes in taste
- difficulty eating and swallowing food

Chronic GVHD in the mouth is usually treated with:

- a topical steroid gel or cream such as fluocinonide or clobetasol gel
- an oral rinse containing dexamethasone, budesonide or prednisolone
- tacrolimus either as a rinse or topical ointment
- pilocarpine (Salagen®) and cevimeline (Evoxac®) for dry mouth

Medications such as lidocaine may be prescribed to control pain.

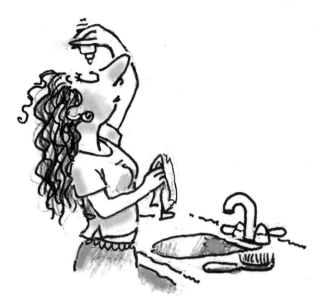

Your Eyes and Chronic GVHD

Chronic GVHD can affect your eyes. Symptoms include:

- dry eyes
- irritation, redness and pain
- sensitivity to bright light or wind
- an inflamed eyelid
- scarring of the eye surface under the lids
- excessive tears

The treatment for GVHD in the eyes depends on the severity of the symptoms. Most cases can be managed with:

- preservative-free artificial tear drops or ointments (preservatives in eye drops can be toxic to eye tissues if used more than 3x per day)
- steroid drops or ointments
- cyclosporine eye drops
- plugging tear ducts so that moisture remains in your eyes
- adding humidity to your home
- wearing goggles to limit exposure to wind

If the problem is more severe and is affecting your vision, your doctor may recommend:

- eye drops made from your blood serum (autologous serum tears)
- a bandage contact lens to protect the surface of the eye
- a scleral contact lens, such as the PROSE system offered by BostonSight®, which has relieved symptoms and improved vision for many patients with severe ocular GVHD

Your Gastrointestinal Tract and Chronic GVHD

Chronic GVHD can affect the esophagus, stomach and colon. Symptoms may include:

- difficult or painful swallowing
- weight loss
- nausea, vomiting and diarrhea

If chronic GVHD affects your gastrointestinal tract, your doctor may recommend treatment with drugs that suppress the immune system or medications that coat the gastrointestinal tract with steroids without affecting other parts of your body. Extracorporeal photopheresis may also help control symptoms.

Your Liver and Chronic GVHD

Chronic GVHD sometimes affects the liver. Symptoms include:

- elevated liver enzyme levels
- jaundice (yellowing of skin and eyes)
- dark urine

If you are diagnosed with chronic GVHD of the liver, your doctor may recommend treatment with:

- prednisone
- tacrolimus
- ursodeoxycholic acid
- extracorporeal photopheresis

Your Lungs and Chronic GVHD

Chronic GVHD sometimes affects the airway passages in the lungs, causing:

- shortness of breath
- wheezing
- coughing

Patients with lung GVHD often do not have any symptoms until the disease has progressed to a serious stage.

If you have GVHD in your lungs, your doctor may treat you with:

- steroid inhalers
- bronchodilators
- tacrolimus
- extracorporeal photopheresis
- montelukast
- azithromycin

Periodic pulmonary function tests are the best way to catch lung GVHD early and begin treatment before you have symptoms.

Your Genitals and Chronic GVHD

Sometimes, chronic GVHD affects the genitals. In women, chronic GVHD can cause:

- dryness, itching, ulcers and scarring in the vagina and on the external genital area
- pain with sex
- pain when urinating

Treatment options may include:

- water based lubricants
- topical steroids

- tacrolimus or cyclosporine ointments
- vaginal suppositories
- dilators to expand the vaginal canal

In men, chronic GVHD may cause itching or scarring on the penis and scrotum. Topical steroids and tacrolimus are the usual treatment options.

Your Nervous System and Chronic GVHD

In rare cases, chronic GVHD can affect the nervous system. Symptoms may include:

- numbness or a painful, tingling sensation in your hands and feet
- shooting pains in your hands and feet
- lack of coordination

These problems, caused by nerve damage, are called neuropathy. Depending on the severity, neuropathy may be treated with:

- topical medications such as a lidocaine patch or gel
- oral medications such as amitriptyline, gabapentin or pregabalin
- physical and occupational therapy
- massage therapy

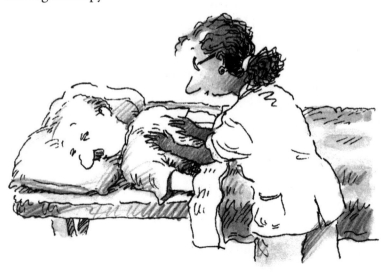

- soaking feet in cool water
- acupuncture

Talk to your doctor if you have symptoms of neuropathy. A consultation with a neurologist can help determine the best treatment for you.

Take care of your feet:

- Wash your feet daily with lukewarm water and fragrance-free soap.
- Inspect your feet daily for cuts, bruises, cracking or other changes that may require attention.
- Wear sturdy shoes or slipper at all times.
- Do not apply direct heat to your feet and legs.

Avoid falls:

- Keep your living area free of clutter and slippery surfaces.
- Consider using devices such as hand rails, canes, etc. to help maintain your balance.

Your Muscles and Chronic GVHD

In rare cases, chronic GVHD may cause muscle weakness. Drugs that suppress the immune system may be used to control this problem.

Other Rare Symptoms of Chronic GVHD

Very rarely, chronic GVHD may cause other symptoms including:

- Raynaud's Phenomenon (poor blood flow to skin, fingers and toes)
- extra fluid around the heart or lungs
- an abnormal accumulation of fluid in the belly
- too much protein in your urine, caused by a kidney problem

Your doctor will rule out other, more common, causes of these symptoms before concluding they are caused by chronic GVHD.

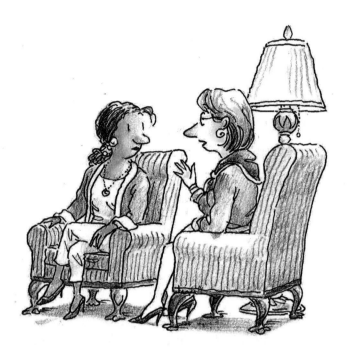

Coping with the Stress of Chronic GVHD

Living with GVHD can be an emotionally difficult experience for both you and your family. After transplant, everyone wants to resume a normal life, but GVHD can make that difficult or impossible for a time.

It's normal to feel sad or anxious while dealing with GVHD. Physical changes, some of the drugs used to treat GVHD, fatigue or insufficient sleep can cause depression, confusion, anxiety, mood swings or exaggerated feelings of anger, excitement or sadness.

Sometimes medications are offered to GVHD patients to stabilize mood swings and reduce anxiety. This is very common, and short-term use of these drugs does not mean you will be dependent on them long-term.

If you have GVHD, it's important not to ignore or downplay your feelings. Finding an outlet to express your feelings can decrease your stress and help you move forward in a healthy manner. This is true for both the patient and caregiver alike.

Talking with a therapist – a social worker, psychologist, psychiatrist or pastoral counselor often helps. Therapists are trained to help you think about problems in a different way so that you can take control of the problem, rather than let the problem control you.

Ask your transplant center or a local hospital for a referral to a therapist in your area who is experienced in helping patients cope with issues like GVHD.

Be The Match® offers free telephone counseling to GVHD patients and their caregivers. Phone 888-999-6743 for details.

Some people find talking one-on-one with another transplant survivor or caregiver helps. BMT InfoNet's Caring Connections Program can put you in touch with others who had GVHD and have experienced the same emotional highs and lows you now face. You can request a Caring Connection online at bmtinfonet.org/caring-connection or by phoning 888-597-7674.

For more information go to our website at:

bmtinfonet.org/gvhd

Chapter Eleven
INFECTION

Six months after my transplant I developed a herpes zoster infection, also known as shingles. I was hospitalized for ten days. That was hard. I was just getting back on my feet and wham! — I'm back in the hospital again.
Marilyn, 11-year transplant survivor

The air we breathe, the food we eat, the items we touch — all the things we come in contact with in daily life are a potential source of bacteria, viruses or fungi that can cause infection. For a healthy individual these daily encounters with sources of infection are not a major problem. Our immune system protects us.

For transplant recipients, however, it's a different story. The high-dose chemotherapy and/or radiation given prior to transplant cannot distinguish between diseased and normal cells. Not only are diseased cells destroyed, but your immune system will be disrupted as well.

Your white blood cell count will be low. Neutrophils, the type of white blood cells that are very helpful in fighting bacterial and fungal infection, will be very low early after transplant – a condition called neutropenia. Other types of white blood cells, called lymphocytes, can take months to recover. Lymphocytes help the body fight viruses and fungi.

Special proteins, called antibodies, that normally help destroy bacteria and viruses are depleted. Until the transplanted stem cells begin producing new white blood cells, you will be extremely vulnerable to infection.

Skin and mucous membranes (lining of the mouth, nose and intestines), which are the body's first line of defense against infection, may also be damaged.

> The first two-to-four weeks after a transplant is a particularly critical time. Although the risk of infection steadily declines once the stem cells begin producing new white blood cells, your immune system does not completely recover and function normally for six months to a year after transplant, and longer if graft-versus-host disease occurs.

The risk of developing a serious bacterial infection is less if you undergo a reduced intensity transplant. This is because the period of neutropenia is often shorter and less severe. The risk for viral and fungal infections are similar between the full intensity and reduced intensity transplants.

Although post-transplant infections are a serious cause for concern, great strides have been made to better manage and prevent them.

Bacterial Infections

Bacteria are microscopic organisms that invade tissues and multiply rapidly. Bacteria can cause infections anywhere in the body and are the usual cause of ear and sinus infections, as well as bronchitis in the lungs.

Bacteria secrete poisonous chemicals called toxins that interfere with normal organ functions. Toxins can cause shock or low blood pressure that can lead to death if sufficient oxygen is not provided to the heart or brain.

Bacteria can also disrupt normal organ functions by their sheer number. Some pneumonias, for example, are caused by rapidly multiplying bacteria that fill up the spaces in your lungs where air is normally absorbed into the body.

Bacterial infections are most common during the first two-to-four weeks following your transplant. The infections occur most often in the intestines, on the skin, and in the mouth. They also occasionally occur in the bladder or lungs.

To combat bacterial infections, antibiotics are usually given during the first few weeks after transplant if your temperature rises above 100.5°F. You may also receive an oral antibiotic before you develop a fever to try to prevent an infection.

To reduce the risk of bacterial infections:

- You should bathe or shower daily to remove bacteria from your skin.

- Use soft toothbrushes or sponges to clean your gums and teeth so that cuts, through which bacteria, fungi and viruses may enter the body, can be avoided.

- Hospital staff and other persons who come in contact with you should carefully wash their hands with antiseptic soap or alcohol based hand sanitizer prior to touching you, since hands are a primary carrier of infectious agents.

- Flowers and plants (both live and dried) which can harbor bacteria or fungi may not be permitted in the room while your immune system is weak.

- Fresh fruits and vegetables or other food items that may increase the risk for food borne infections may be eliminated from your diet until your immune system is functioning normally.

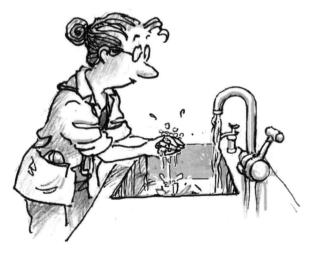

When detected promptly and treated with antibiotics, bacterial infections are usually well managed.

Fungal Infections

Fungi are primitive life forms that we encounter daily. Bread mold is an example of a common fungus. Most are harmless and some, such as the fungus called Candida, normally reside inside our body.

Fungal infections are less common than bacterial infections in the first few weeks after transplant but are very difficult to treat. Unfortunately, while the widespread use of antibiotics after transplant has successfully reduced the incidence of harmful bacterial infections, those antibiotics can also destroy beneficial bacteria in the body that keep fungi in check.

At some transplant centers:

- special air filtering equipment is installed in patient hospital rooms to remove fungi from the air
- fresh plants, fruits and vegetables are removed from the patient's environment to reduce the risk of fungal infections
- patients are given an anti-fungal medication to prevent fungal infection early after transplant
- patients who have continuous fevers after taking antibiotics may receive a different anti-fungal drug to control the development of fungal infections

Candida and aspergillus are the most common fungal infections after transplant. Candida lives in the intestines, mouth and vagina and is normally kept in check by bacteria. When bacteria are destroyed by antibiotics, however, the fungi can multiply and spread, infecting many parts of the body. A drug called fluconazole may be used to control Candida infections.

Aspergillus infections occur most often in the sinus passages or lungs, and can cause pneumonia. The aspergillus fungus is frequently found around construction sites or where buildings are being remodeled. It has also been identified in marijuana and is not killed by burning or cooking marijuana. Voriconazole, posocanasole and isavuconazonium sulfate are effective in treating aspergillus infections.

A fungus called pneumocystis jirovecii (formerly called pneumocystis carinii) is found in the trachea (windpipe) of healthy humans. When a person's immune system is suppressed, this fungus can enter the lungs and grow into tiny cysts which can cause pneumonia. Trimethoprim/sulfamethoxazole (Bactrim® or Septra®) atovaqone, dapsone and pentamidine are effective in preventing and treating pneumocystis jiroveci pneumonia.

Once your blood counts return to normal levels, the risk of fungal infection drops dramatically.

Viral Infections

Viruses are tiny parasites that invade other organisms, such as human cells, in order to survive. Viruses tinker with the genetic machinery of the host cell, turning it into a factory for the production of more of the virus. The virus eventually destroys or cripples the host cell and moves on to neighboring cells to continue the process.

Infections caused by viruses are very difficult to treat. Several antiviral agents such as acyclovir and ganciclovir are useful, but the number of viruses they effectively treat is small. Viral infections

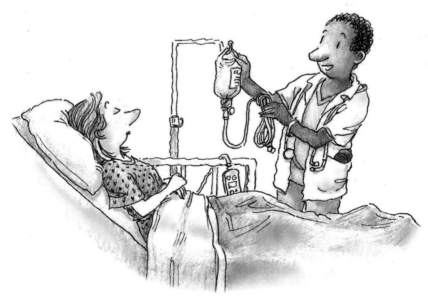

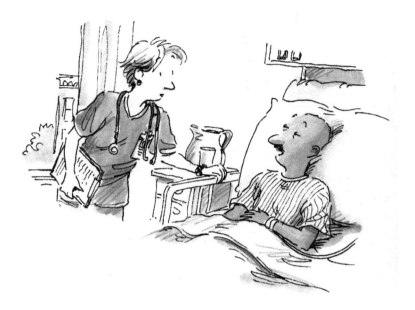

following transplant occur either as a result of exposure to a new virus or reactivation of an old virus that was already in your body.

The viral infections that occur most often following transplant are caused by the herpes simplex virus (HSV), varicella zoster virus (VZV) or cytomegalovirus (CMV).

Herpes Simplex (HSV)

Herpes simplex infections are caused by two separate viruses: herpes I and herpes II. Herpes I causes painful fever blisters in and around the mouth. Herpes II causes painful blisters on the genitalia and/or rectum.

An estimated 70 percent of Americans are exposed to the herpes I virus, usually during childhood. The virus is highly contagious and is usually transmitted through contact with people who have active herpes sores on their mouth.

Herpes II, on the other hand, is usually transmitted through sexual intercourse with an infected partner.

Herpes infections often recur after the initial episode. The virus can lay dormant in the body for many years, flaring up from time-to-time.

Herpes infections usually occur during the first month after transplant. Herpes simplex responds well to treatment with anti-viral agents such as acyclovir. Most centers give patients acyclovir before a herpes infection develops which has greatly reduced the incidence of herpes infections after transplant.

Varicella Zoster Virus (VZV)

Varicella zoster virus is often referred to as herpes zoster or shingles. It is the same virus that causes chicken pox. VZV is seen most often in patients being treated for leukemia, lymphoma or Hodgkin disease.

VZV infections can cause an itching, blistering skin rash that extends along any one of the body's nerve branches. The nerve endings under the skin at the site of the rash are infected and can cause great pain.

A VZV infection can also develop in the nerve to the eye called the ophthalmic nerve. A painful rash may occur along the nerve path on the forehead and eyelids. If not treated promptly the infection can damage the eye.

VZV infections may be treated with oral doses of famciclovir or valcyclovir, or acyclovir given intravenously. They are quite contagious and some patients must be admitted to the hospital to be treated.

> The pain associated with a VZV infection can be significantly reduced if you call your doctor the day the rash first appears. Medications such as acetaminophen, codeine or morphine may be administered to control pain. Early treatment can significantly reduce the duration of VZV infections.

A VZV infection can occur more than once after transplant. The itching and pain associated with a VZV infection can continue long after all clinical signs of the disease disappear. Some patients require prolonged use of medications to treat the nerve pain from a VZV infection.

Since VZV infections are highly contagious, patients should avoid people with chicken pox or a VZV infection for the first year after transplant.

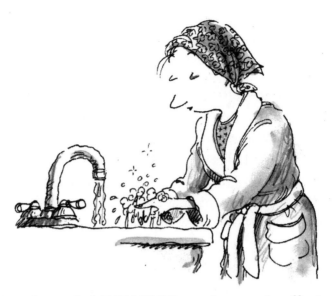

Recently, a drug called SHINGRIX® was shown to be effective in preventing zoster infections in patients. This vaccine series can start as early as two months after transplant. The other available VZV vaccine, Zostavax®, should not be given until two years after transplant.

Cytomegalovirus (CMV)

CMV infections can develop in different organs including the liver, colon, eyes or lungs. Although all CMV infections are cause for concern, CMV pneumonia is particularly worrisome because it is difficult to treat. You may be given letermovir to prevent a CMV infection.

Some patients who are very high risk are given ganciclovir to prevent CMV infections. However, most patients are monitored for signs of the virus in the blood and then started on treatment.

Approximately 60 percent of the general population is exposed to CMV during their lifetime, particularly urban dwellers. Doctors can test your blood prior to transplant to determine whether or not CMV is present in your body. If it is not, care will be taken to prevent exposure to CMV before, during and after the transplant.

Filtering blood transfusions given to you to remove most of the white blood cells reduces your risk of developing a CMV infection.

Other Viruses

Common viruses, such as those that cause a cold (rhinovirus, coronavirus, parainfluenza virus) or the influenza virus can cause serious infections for patients up to a year after transplant. Other viruses such as adenovirus, papovavirus, Epstein-Barr virus (EBV), respiratory syncytial virus (RSV) and human papilloma virus (HPV) can also create problems post-transplant, although the incidence of these infections is quite low.

Adenovirus and RSV infections can cause pneumonia. Adenovirus can also cause an infection in the kidneys or gastrointestinal tract. Ribavirin is effective in treating both of these viruses.

The likelihood of developing these viral infections can be greatly reduced by limiting contact with the public after transplant (particularly people with the flu or a cold) and by meticulous hand washing. Some centers require a brief period of isolation from the general public after transplant to reduce the risk of getting one of these viruses.

Protozoa

Protozoa are single-cell parasites that feed on organisms such as human cells to survive. Although infections from protozoa are less common than bacterial or viral infections, they can pose serious problems for transplant patients.

An infection called toxoplasmosis occasionally develops after transplant. Toxoplasmosis is caused by a protozoan called toxoplasma gondii which is often transmitted in the feces of cats. Toxoplasmosis may infect the brain, eyes, muscles, liver and/or lungs. A painful inflamed eye retina is a common manifestation of the disease which, without prompt treatment, can result in damage to your eyes. With early diagnosis and proper treatment, toxoplasmosis is treatable.

Preventing Infection

Although it may be tempting to throw caution to the wind after your stem cell transplant, it's best not to take chances. Bacteria, viruses and fungi that are harmless to most people can cause very serious infections until your immune system has fully recovered.

Your medical team will give you guidelines to help prevent infections. The most important of these is frequent hand washing with antibacterial soap and water or an alcohol-based hand sanitizer, especially before eating or preparing food and after:

- changing diapers (if you are permitted to do so)
- touching plants or dirt (if you are permitted to do so)
- going to the bathroom
- touching animals
- touching bodily fluids or items that might have come in contact with bodily fluids such as clothing, bedding or toilets
- going outdoors or to a public place
- removing gloves
- collecting or depositing garbage (if you are permitted to do so)
- before and after touching catheters and wounds

During the first six months after your transplant, and longer if you take immunosuppressive drugs, your transplant center may recommend that you avoid:

- crowds or people who have infections
- people who have recently been vaccinated with chicken pox or polio
- changing a baby's diapers
- gardening
- walking, wading, swimming or playing in ponds or lakes
- construction sites and remodeling projects
- well water that has not been treated

If You Have Pets

Rules vary among transplant centers as to whether or not you can have pets in the home while you are recovering. Consult your transplant center for its guidelines.

Your transplant team may advise you to avoid:

- contact with an animal that is ill
- adopting ill or juvenile pets (juvenile pets are more likely to scratch than mature pets)
- reptiles such as lizards, snakes, turtles and iguanas and items they touch
- chicks and ducklings
- exotic pets such as monkeys or chinchillas

Your transplant team may also advise you to:

- feed pets only high quality commercial food or thoroughly cooked human food
- not clean litter boxes or cages or dispose of animal waste
- not touch bird droppings
- avoid cleaning fish tanks
- not place cat litter boxes in areas of the house where food is prepared or eaten
- keep cats indoors and not adopt stray cats
- cover backyard sandboxes to prevent cats from using it as a litter box

At the first sign of fever or infection, call your physician. Infections are most easily treated when caught early. Infections you formerly ignored can be serious problems after transplant. Taking precautions to guard against infection can be a nuisance, but it can also save your life.

Re-vaccination

After a stem cell transplant, it is likely that antibodies provided by previous vaccines may be lost or depleted. Guidelines developed by transplant specialists and available for viewing on the Centers for Disease Control website suggest that patients may need to be re-vaccinated for diphtheria, tetanus, pneumococcus, hemophilus, influenza type B and polio infections beginning six-to-18 months after transplant. The guidelines recommend waiting until at least two years after transplant to receive the MMR vaccine for measles, mumps, and rubella.

Your transplant team may recommend that you get the flu vaccine starting at six months after transplant. Discuss this issue with your transplant doctor to determine appropriate timing of re-vaccinations for you.

For more information go to our website at:

bmtinfonet.org/prevent-infection

Chapter Twelve
NUTRITION

After my transplant, I was the nausea queen. You name it, I could throw it up. For a while, all I could handle was Carnation Instant Breakfast®. Then I worked my way up to Cap'n Crunch®— box after box of it — then coffee and beer, and finally, at long last, a normal diet.

Judith, six-year transplant survivor

We all need food and water to thrive. The calories in food provide the fuel your organs and tissues need to grow and function. Protein-rich foods enable your body to build and repair muscle and body tissue. Vitamins and minerals keep your blood, skin and nervous system functioning properly.

Transplant patients have unique nutritional requirements. Prior to transplant, you will undergo high-dose chemotherapy and/or total body irradiation (TBI) to destroy your disease. This severely stresses your body's organs and tissues. In order to repair any organ or tissue damage that might occur and to fight fever, you will need to increase your intake of calories and protein.

Transplant patients typically require 50-60 percent more calories and twice as much protein in their diet than healthy individuals of similar age and gender. This need for more calories and protein usually persists at least one-to-two months after transplant.

Changing Diet before Transplant

Some patients consider making major dietary changes before transplant. Some attempt to shed excess weight or increase their intake of foods that have been associated with a lower incidence of cancer. Others turn to macrobiotic or other diets that restrict the types of foods you consume.

If you are considering changing your diet, ask your doctor for a referral to a registered dietitian who can evaluate the nutritional adequacy of your new diet. Some diets, such as macrobiotic diets, contain lower amounts of protein and other nutrients than are required by a recovering transplant patient.

Using certain herbs, roots or dietary supplements can be dangerous for you while you're undergoing transplantation. Consult your doctor or dietitian before using these products.

Quick weight loss is also usually discouraged. Since you will likely lose weight while undergoing treatment, limiting food intake before your transplant could cause a serious nutrient deficiency.

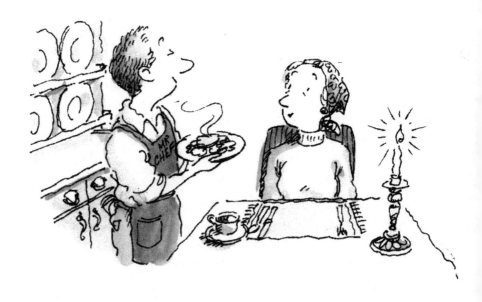

Several studies have suggested a relationship between types of foods consumed and the risk of developing cancer. However, no study has proven that changing your diet can cure cancer.

Nutrition after Transplant

For the first three months after transplant, or longer if you are taking immunosuppressive drugs, you will be advised to avoid foods that may contain organisms that could cause infection. Many transplant centers have specific recommendations on foods to avoid which may include:

- raw or undercooked meat
- dishes that contain undercooked meat
- raw or undercooked eggs, or foods that might contain them
- raw or undercooked seafood such as sushi
- raw nuts or unshelled nuts that are not roasted
- meats and cheese from a deli
- miso and tempeh products
- milk products that are not pasteurized including Mexican-style soft cheese such as queso fresco and queso blanco
- cheeses with mold such as blue cheese, Brie, Camembert, Gorgonzola, Roquefort and Stilton
- soft cheeses such as feta, goat cheese and farmer's cheese
- smoked, uncooked refrigerated fish such as nova lox
- pickled seafood
- raw honey
- salad bars and buffets

Some transplant centers include fresh fruits and vegetables on the list of foods to avoid, while others permit them provided they are thoroughly washed. Consult your transplant team to learn which dietary restrictions apply to you and for how long.

Consuming sufficient calories, protein and fluids can be difficult particularly during the first few weeks after transplant. Mouth sores, nausea, vomiting, dry mouth, diarrhea, constipation, depression and fatigue can make mealtimes unappealing. Certain medications can also cause a loss of appetite.

Some patients must be fed intravenously during this period to ensure they receive sufficient calories, protein, vitamins, minerals and fluids. The intravenous feeding is called total parenteral nutrition (TPN) or hyperalimentation and may supply all your nutritional requirements or supplement those you are able to consume on your own.

Often, eating problems can be overcome without resorting to the use of TPN. The following sections describe common eating problems after transplant and suggestions for overcoming them.

Mouth and Throat Sores

Mouth and throat sores are common after transplant. They may be caused by chemotherapy, total body irradiation or infection. If mouth sores are a problem for you try:

- lukewarm or cold food, rather than hot food
- cooking foods until tender and soft
- drinking through a straw to bypass mouth sores
- high-protein, high-calorie foods to speed healing of the sores
- a liquid or blenderized diet, or a complete nutrition supplement such as Ensure®, Boost®, or Carnation Instant Breakfast®
- soft foods such as creamed soups, pasteurized cheese, mashed potatoes, cooked eggs, custards, puddings, gelatin, canned fruit cooked cereals and pasteurized eggnog
- cold foods such as milk shakes, ice cream, cottage cheese, yogurt, watermelon, and slushes
- soft, frozen foods such as popsicles, ice cream and frozen yogurt
- pasteurized fruit nectars and fruit flavored beverages instead of acidic juices

If you develop mouth or throat sores, avoid:

- tart or acidic foods and beverages such as citrus fruits and juices, pineapple juice and tomato products
- salty foods, including broth
- strong spices such as peppers, chili powder, nutmeg and cloves
- coarse foods such as raw fruits and vegetables, dry toast, grainy cereals and breads, and crunchy snacks
- alcoholic beverages and mouthwashes that contain alcohol
- extremely hot foods or beverages

If your mouth pain is severe, ask your transplant team for pain medication.

Dry Mouth

Dry mouth is a common side effect of total body irradiation, anti-nausea medications and antihistamines. If a dry mouth is making eating difficult, try the following:

- Add sauces, gravies, broth and dressings to foods.
- Suck ice chips, popsicles, sugarless gum or hard candies to keep your mouth moist.
- Add citric acid to your diet to stimulate saliva production, unless you have mouth or throat sores. Citric acid is present in oranges, orange juice, lemons, lemonade and sugarless lemon drops. You can also add lemon to tea, water and soda.
- Drink liquids with your meals.
- Ask your dietitian or doctor about commercial saliva substitutes such as Salivart®, Mouth-Kote®, and Bioténe®.

Avoid eating:

- meats without sauces
- bread products, crackers and dry cakes
- very hot food and beverages
- alcoholic beverages and mouthwashes that contain alcohol

Changes in Taste

Total body irradiation, chemotherapy and some pain medications can make foods you normally enjoy taste unpleasant. To overcome this problem, try eating or drinking:

- cold foods and beverages

- strongly flavored foods such as chocolate, lasagna, spaghetti or barbequed foods, unless you also have mouth or throat sores

- tart or spicy foods, unless you also have mouth or throat sores

- fluids with your meal to rinse away any bad taste

- high-protein foods without strong odors, such as poultry, eggs, and dairy products rather than those with strong odors such as beef and fish

- sauces with foods

- meat with something sweet, such as cranberry sauce, jelly or applesauce

- new seasoning combinations or adding sugar or salt to enhance the taste

Select foods that smell appetizing. If food has a metallic taste, try using plastic eating utensils.

Thick Saliva

Total body irradiation and dehydration can cause thick saliva. If thick saliva is making eating difficult, try the following:

- Drink club soda (seltzer) or hot tea with lemon.

- Suck sugarless sour lemon drops.

- Eat a lighter breakfast if you have mucous build up in the morning, and bigger meals in the afternoon and evening.

- Rinse frequently with a saline solution (one quart water with 1/2-to-3/4 teaspoons salt, and one-to-two teaspoons baking soda).

- Drink lots of fluids.

- Eat soft, tender foods such as cooked fish and chicken, eggs, noodles, hot cereals thinned with water, blenderized fruits and vegetables diluted to a very thin consistency.
- Eat small, frequent meals.
- Drink diluted juices, broth-based soups, and fruit-flavored beverages.
- Switch to a liquid diet if the problem is severe.

Avoid eating:

- meats that require chewing
- bread products
- oily foods
- thick cream soups
- thick hot cereals
- nectars

Nausea and Vomiting

High-dose chemotherapy, total body irradiation, infections and drugs used to control infections, opioid medications, interferon, and mucous drainage from your mouth and sinuses can trigger nausea and vomiting.

If nausea and vomiting are interfering with your ability to eat, try eating:

- small frequent meals
- dry crackers or toast, especially before movement, such as getting out of bed, unless you have mouth sores
- cold foods, rather than warm foods, because they tend to have less food odor
- low-fat foods such as cooked vegetables, canned fruit, baked skinless chicken, sherbet, fruit ice, popsicles, gelatin, pretzels, vanilla wafers and angel food cake

- clear, cool liquids such as carbonated beverages, flavored gelatin, popsicles and ice cubes made of a favorite liquid
- liquids sipped slowly through a straw
- small amounts of liquid frequently throughout the day

Ask for medication to control nausea if it is severe.

If you're hospitalized, you can:

- request anti-nausea medication 30 minutes before your meal
- ask that food trays be brought to you without covers on the plates to avoid being overwhelmed by the smell when the cover is removed

Avoid eating or drinking:

- spicy food
- foods that are overly sweet
- strong smelling foods
- foods that are high in fat
- hot liquids with meals
- liquids if you have an empty stomach

If you are nauseated, avoid lying flat on your back after eating. This can make the problem worse. If you need rest, sit or recline with your head elevated.

Avoid perfumes and other strong smelling cosmetics.

Lack of Appetite/Weight Loss

Many transplant patients experience weight loss and lack of appetite for a period of time. Possible causes include total body irradiation, chemotherapy, infection, depression and fatigue. If you have no appetite for food following your transplant try eating:

- small frequent high-calorie meals.
- high-nutrient liquids such as juice or milk instead of low-calorie drinks like coffee, tea or diet soda.

- nutrient-dense, high-calorie foods like:
  - pasteurized cheese, whole milk and ice cream
  - eggs
  - avocados
  - olives
  - Greek yogurt
  - hummus
  - trail mix
  - fruit smoothies
  - protein powder added to food or drinks
  - dried fruit
  - peanut butter
  - wheat germ
  - nuts
  - fruits
- protein supplements such ProMod® or complete nutrition supplements such as Ensure®, Boost®, Carnation Instant Breakfast® or Sustacal®, provided they have been approved by your dietitian.
- non-fat dry milk powder added to casseroles, cooked cereals and mixed dishes.

You can also try:

- creating a pleasant, mealtime atmosphere, such as colorful place settings, varied food colors and textures, soft music
- light exercise to stimulate your appetite
- addressing any psychological problems that may be causing loss of appetite
- asking your doctor about medications that can improve your appetite

Diarrhea

Diarrhea can occur following total body irradiation or high-dose chemotherapy. It may also be caused by an infection called Clostridium difficile colitis or C. diff, for short.

Some antibiotics and oral medications, such as magnesium salts or metoclopramide (Reglan®) can also cause diarrhea. Diarrhea may be caused by infection or lactose intolerance — an inability to digest the lactose in milk products.

If you are experiencing diarrhea try the eating or drinking:

- smaller amounts of food at each meal
- extra fluids to prevent dehydration
- fluids between meals rather than with meals
- foods and beverages high in potassium such as:
    - ripe bananas
    - potatoes without the skin
    - tomato juice, Gatorade®, Pedialyte®, Powerade®, orange juice and pasteurized peach and pear nectar
    - baked fish and chicken, ground beef
    - well-cooked eggs
    - well-cooked vegetables (but not beans, broccoli, cauliflower or cabbage)
    - canned fruit
    - white rice
    - white bread.

Avoid eating:

- bran, whole grain cereals and bread
- raw vegetables
- fruits with skin and seeds
- popcorn, nuts and seeds
- carbonated beverages

- beans, broccoli, cauliflower and cabbage
- chewing gum
- spicy foods
- foods with rich gravies or sauces
- foods and drinks with caffeine such as coffee, tea, chocolate, colas and other caffeinated drinks
- dairy products, unless they are treated with Lactaid®

Do not take over-the-counter anti-diarrhea medications, like Imodium®, unless approved by your doctor, since these drugs sometimes make a colon infection worse.

Constipation

Some chemotherapy drugs, opioid pain medications and anti-nausea medications cause constipation. Try eating or drinking:

- warm beverages
- high-fiber foods such as well-washed raw fruits and vegetables, whole wheat bread and cereals, dried fruit, dried peas and beans. Be sure you drink plenty of fluids while eating these foods.
- Warm prune juice or stewed prunes

Light exercise may also help with constipation. Ask your doctor about stool softeners or laxatives if the problem persists for more than two days.

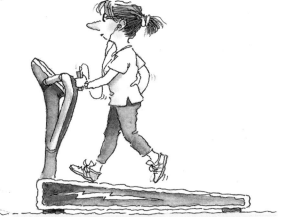

Herbs, Botanicals and Supplements

Until your immune system has fully recovered, you should avoid taking any herb, botanical or supplement without your doctor's approval. Some of these products can:

- reduce the effectiveness of drugs prescribed by your doctor
- cause a serious infection, due to inadequate purification of the product or extra ingredients it contains
- damage your liver, kidneys or other organs
- make gastrointestinal problems worse
- interfere with blood clotting

Herbal and botanical products to avoid while your immune system is recovering include:

- alfalfa
- borage
- chaparral
- Chinese herbs
- coltsfoot
- comfrey
- DHEA
- dieter's tea (including senna, aloe, rhubarb root, buckthorn, cascara and castor oil)
- ephedra or mahuange
- groundsel or life root
- heliotrope or valerian
- kava kava
- laetrile (apricot pits)
- licorice root

- lobelia
- L-tryptophan
- maté tea
- Pau D'Arco
- pennyroyal
- sassafras
- St. John's wort
- yohimbe and yohimbine

If your platelet count is low, you should avoid garlic pill supplements (cooking with regular garlic is fine) and gingko biloba, which can interfere with blood clotting.

Check with your doctor to see whether there are other herbs, supplements or botanicals that you should avoid while your immune system is recovering, or while you are on medications that may interact with them.

Resources

Eating and maintaining your weight is very important after transplant. Most transplant programs have a registered dietician available to help you manage eating difficulties during treatment. If you continue to have eating difficulties long-term, consult the dietician at your transplant center.

To learn more, go to our website at:

bmtinfonet.org/nutrition

Chapter Thirteen
RELIEVING PAIN

I was given a wonderful little button that allowed me to self-dispense morphine every five minutes. I pushed it a lot. I don't remember much more about that week — I've blocked it out. It's a fog and I'm glad.

Jim, five-year transplant survivor

Like many other patients, you may find the prospect of pain more frightening than other potential transplant complications. In this chapter, we'll examine the type of pain transplant recipients sometimes experience and the various drugs used to control it. We'll also discuss some non-drug techniques that can help provide relief.

What is Pain?

Today's pain specialists agree that pain is whatever a patient says it is, wherever, whenever and to whatever degree he or she says it occurs. The sensation of pain is influenced by physical factors such as tissue damage as well as by psychological, social and environmental factors.

Two different people with the same amount of tissue damage may experience very different levels of pain. Moreover, each person's body absorbs and processes pain medications differently. Thus, the amount of medication needed to ease one person's pain may differ greatly from that required to ease another's pain. In short, pain is a very personal experience requiring a highly individualized response from the medical team.

Pain can be described as acute or chronic. Acute pain, usually due to tissue damage, lasts days-to-weeks and ends once the tissue damage is healed. Most pain experienced by transplant patients is acute pain. The word acute does not mean that the pain is sharper or more uncomfortable. It simply refers to the length of time over which pain occurs.

Chronic pain persists over months or years and is caused by irreparable tissue damage, nerve damage, chronic graft-versus-host disease or by unknown causes. Often, chronic pain can only be controlled; its source cannot be eliminated.

How Pain is Experienced

The pain patients experience while undergoing a blood stem cell transplant is usually caused by temporary inflammation of tissues or nerves. Sensors at the tissue or nerve site detect the physical damage and transmit distress signals to the brain.

Suffering is a person's response to those pain signals. The degree of suffering varies greatly depending on your emotional and physical condition at the time pain is experienced. Fatigue, depression, anxiety, physical weakness, memories of how well your pain was managed in the past and fears about the cause of the pain can increase the suffering associated with pain.

Blocking Pain Signals

The sensation of pain is relieved by blocking the pain signals as they travel from the site of the injury to the brain. The signals are blocked with drugs or through a combination of drug and non-drug therapies.

The most commonly used pain medications for transplant patients are opioids. Opioids include drugs such as morphine and hydromorphone (Dilaudid®). Non-opioid drugs such as aspirin, ibuprofen and acetaminophen are often not strong enough to provide sufficient pain relief and may have side effects that can cause problems for transplant patients.

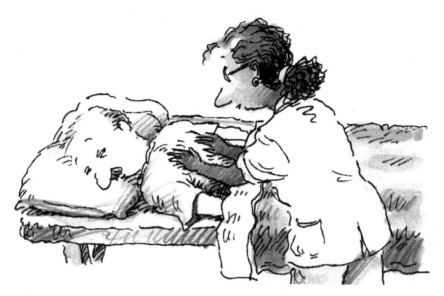

At some transplant centers, massage, application of heat or cold to the affected area, exercise, relaxation, visualization, hypnosis and distraction are used to enhance the relief provided by pain medications.

Pain Common after a Stem Cell Transplant

Each person's transplant experience is unique. Some people experience only mild discomfort and need only small amounts of pain medication. Others experience more significant pain and require more medication to control it.

Mouth and Skin Sores

Painful mouth sores are a frequent side effect of transplantation. Pain medications, such as Lidocaine®, can be used like a mouth wash to control the discomfort. In many cases, an opioid, such as morphine, is given to provide additional relief.

High-dose chemotherapy and radiation can cause skin sores. Opioids are typically used to control the pain. If a burning sensation accompanies the pain, aloe vera gel (without an alcohol base), Eucerin® or Silvaderm™/Lidocaine® cream may be applied directly to the skin.

Medical Procedures

Certain medical procedures can cause temporary discomfort. A bone marrow aspirate is a good example. In this procedure, a needle is inserted into the rear hip bone to withdraw a sample of bone marrow. While the area around the bone can be numbed, it's not possible to numb the bone itself. An uncomfortable scraping sensation and pressure are common with bone marrow aspirates.

Anxiety about the procedure can be reduced by pre-medicating you with a small amount of Versed® or Ativan® to relax you, and a small dosage of opioid to help relieve the pain. Don't be embarrassed to ask for pre-medication to ease your anxiety if you're fearful about a bone marrow aspirate.

In some cases, it may be possible for your healthcare team to briefly sedate you with powerful, short-term general anesthetics, in addition to local anesthetics, so that you are not fully conscious while the procedure is taking place. This technique, called conscious sedation, requires an anesthesiologist and more elaborate preparation, such as withholding food and drink for six to seven hours prior to the procedure. If you are anxious about painful medical procedures, inquire about this technique.

Growth Factors

Growth factors given to patients to speed the recovery of bone marrow after transplant can cause mild to moderate bone pain, muscle pain and/or headaches. In most cases, the pain can be controlled with acetaminophen or an antihistamine such as Claritin® and ends when you stop taking growth factors. If the pain is severe, opioids may be used to relieve it.

Infections

Infections may cause mild, moderate or severe pain. Opioids are not effective in eliminating infection-related pain, but can help control the pain while the antibiotic or anti-fungal drug begins to work. If an infection develops after you are discharged from the hospital, you may need to be hospitalized for several days to quickly bring the infection and pain under control.

Graft-versus-Host Disease

If you develop graft-versus-host disease (GVHD) you may develop a painful skin rash. You may also experience heartburn, stomach pain and/or a burning sensation when eating acidic foods. Opioids are useful for controlling pain caused by GVHD. Benadryl® or topical hydrocortisone cream may help relieve the itching associated with skin GVHD. Bentyl® and Lomotil® may relieve cramping caused by intestinal GVHD.

Neuropathy

Neuropathy is a nerve condition that sometimes occurs after transplant. Neuropathy can cause pain or tingling in the hands and feet. The discomfort may be greater at night or in cold weather.

If you are experiencing symptoms of neuropathy, consult a neurologist. The neurologist will conduct a thorough examination to determine what type of neuropathy you are experiencing so that it can be properly treated.

Although it is not possible to cure the nerve damage that causes neuropathy, several drugs are available to treat the associated pain. Non-drug therapies such as transcutaneous electrical nerve stimulation (TENS), biofeedback and hypnosis may also help.

You can learn more about managing neuropathy at bmtinfonet.org/neuropathy.

Identify the Cause of Pain

In order to properly treat pain, its cause must be identified. Most pain has a physical cause that can either be seen by a physician or deduced based on the patient's history and description of the pain.

> Notify your physician or nurse about pain as soon as it begins. It is easier to relieve pain in the early stages than after it has become severe. There is no need to endure pain, and no reason to be embarrassed about asking for relief. In fact, refusing pain medication may be harmful. Patients who are gripped by pain are often less able to do important things that are necessary for recovery, such as eating or exercising.

Sometimes a physical cause for the pain is not readily apparent. This does not mean that the pain is any less real or less urgent to relieve. Pain experts agree that when you say that you are experiencing pain, it's important for your healthcare team to take that complaint seriously and attempt to relieve it, whether or not a physical cause is apparent.

You can help your physician properly identify the cause of pain by being very specific about the description, intensity, location and frequency of the pain.

Rate the pain on a scale of 0-10 (0=no pain, 10=worst pain).

- Is it mild, moderate or severe?
- Is it sharp or a dull ache? Does it throb? Is there a burning or itching sensation associated with it?
- Is it constant or intermittent? If it's intermittent, how often does it occur?
- How long does it last?
- Is it better or worse at certain times of the day or night?
- When did it begin?
- Do certain actions or motions such as lying down or taking a deep breath make the pain better or worse?
- How is it affecting your daily life?

The more information the physician has about the pain, the more likely he or she will be able to identify and treat both the cause and symptoms properly.

Choosing a Drug and Dosage

The drug chosen to relieve pain will depend on the physical cause of the pain. Opioids are effective in controlling pain from tissue damage, such as mouth sores or skin rashes, but may be less effective in controlling pain associated with nerve irritation, such as that caused by herpes zoster. Anti-depressants and anti-convulsants may help control pain caused by nerve damage.

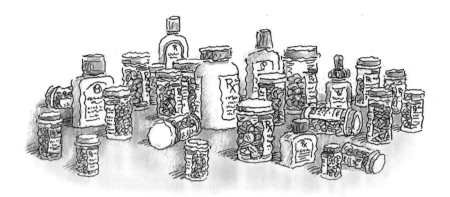

> The dosage of medication required to relieve pain varies considerably among patients. There is nothing wrong with you if you require more medication to relieve pain. Each person's body reacts differently to pain medications.

Some drugs are very slow acting but produce long-term pain relief. Others quickly reduce pain but are effective only for a short period of time. A combination of drugs is sometimes used to provide patients with the best relief.

Maintaining Relief

If your pain increases, the dosage of a drug needed to relieve the pain may also need to be increased. Some drugs, such as opioids, provide additional pain relief whenever the dosage is increased, while others do not.

Increasing the dosage of drugs may increase the risk of side effects. These side effects are usually minor and reversible, but you should not increase the dosage or frequency of pain medications without first checking with your doctor.

While in the hospital or clinic, nurses may administer pain medications or you may be given a Patient Controlled Analgesia machine (PCA) that allows you to administer your own pain medication, up to a safe limit, as needed. The PCA can be adjusted to dispense pain medication during periods when you are sleeping.

Pain relief may also be administered by a pain patch applied to the skin that delivers narcotics continuously for three days.

Fear of Addiction

Most patients undergoing transplantation require pain medications at some point. One of the biggest barriers to providing patients with adequate pain relief is the fear of addiction. Thus, some opt to put up with pain rather than ask for pain medication.

Pain medication will be given to you only as long as you need it. Your care team will taper down the dosage once your pain is under control. Unless you have a history of drug or alcohol addiction, it is unlikely that you will become addicted to pain medications.

What if Pain Continues?

Since pain relief must be tailored to your individual needs, it may take some time before the appropriate type and level of pain medication can be determined. You can help your doctor by providing feedback on how well the pain medications are working.

- Has the medication provided any relief at all?
- Does the drug wear off before you're scheduled to take the next dosage?
- Are you experiencing any side effects such as drowsiness, nervousness, nausea, itching or constipation?

When you are given pain medication, ask when you can expect it to take effect. While you're waiting for it to work, try to find a distraction from the pain. If the drug fails to relieve the pain when expected, notify your doctor or nurse. He or she will adjust the dosage or change your prescription until pain relief is achieved.

If you feel you are not receiving adequate pain relief, talk to your doctor or ask a family member to raise this problem with the doctors and nurses. Spouses, parents and other caregivers can be very effective advocates for pain relief, particularly if you are too exhausted or embarrassed to seek help on your own.

Non-Drug Pain Control Techniques

Olympic athletes do it. Football stars do it. In fact everyone, at some time or another, has relied on methods to relieve discomfort that don't involve drugs.

When a child falls and bruises himself, for example, a parent may show him an interesting toy to take his attention away from the pain. Women preparing for childbirth often take prenatal classes that teach them how to use breathing exercises to relieve pain during labor and delivery. Heat, cold, immobilization, or physical therapy are commonly used by athletes to relieve pain caused by sports injuries.

While drugs will be the primary source of pain relief for you, non-drug therapies such as positive coping statements, distraction, relaxation, imagery, hypnosis, application of heat or cold to the affected area, massage and exercise can enhance pain relief.

Positive Coping Statements

Fear and a feeling of helplessness are common among transplant patients. Not only has a powerful disease taken control of your body, but you are forced to rely on a team of complete strangers to save your life. Anger and frustration over this lack of control can lead to anxiety and depression, which in turn can make it more difficult to tolerate pain.

Although these negative thoughts and feelings are normal, you can often exercise some control over them with positive coping statements.

- Focus on the various things you can do rather than those that you can't do.

- Try to take encouragement from even small accomplishments or try to find something positive in each experience.

- If you're discouraged because the days of treatment seem to be passing slowly, try focusing on the fact that you have already successfully made it through several days, and that you are moving closer to the day of full recovery.

If you experience some backsliding, e.g., your blood counts go down or your body is not responding to certain medications, remind yourself that temporary setbacks are normal and not a cause for alarm. Think about the progress you have made overall since starting your treatment and try not to measure each day against the successes of a prior day.

You may find that repeating encouraging phrases such as the words 'I am coping well' helps.

> "I had a friend — an older gentleman — who came to my house before the transplant. He was 6'-4", had a tall crop of white hair, wore cowboy boots, lean jeans and a rope tie. He said he was going to help me relax and keep the pain from my mind. He taught me several relaxation techniques. I was always able to call him and he'd give me some key words or phrases that helped me start relaxing until the medications arrived or until I stopped panicking."

If it is difficult to find something positive in each day's experience, ask the hospital social worker, pastoral counselor, psychologist or psychiatry staff for help. Often they can suggest ways to cope with your frustrations and refocus your attention on more positive thoughts.

Distraction

Distraction is probably the most familiar non-drug pain control technique. Watching a movie, listening to soothing music, or talking with visitors can divert your attention from discomfort and focus it on a more pleasurable experience.

Before your transplant, think about the kinds of activities that will help pass the time and provide a distraction from worry and pain. Set aside

- recordings of music or stories
- movies (with uncomplicated plots)
- books (simple stories or picture books may be all you can handle)
- video or family games that you enjoy

Keep in mind that you'll often be groggy, your attention span will be shorter and your coordination will be temporarily diminished while you're taking medication. Thus, you may not be able to handle the more complicated hobbies or activities you normally enjoy until later.

You may find that conversations with family members or friends are the most helpful distraction from pain. Having a caregiver read to you or simply listening to conversations among visitors can be pleasant.

Storytelling is an excellent distraction for children. Letting the child tell the story with you works best, but listening to stories can be helpful as well. Art projects also work well with children who are usually less inhibited than adults about testing their artistic talents and ideas.

Relaxation and Imagery

Relaxation and imagery are two commonly used techniques to relieve anxiety and pain. Relaxation involves a series of muscle tensing and relaxing exercises or focused breathing exercises that are designed to induce a sense of calm in the body.

Relaxation is most effective when combined with imagery. Imagery involves thinking of a pleasant, safe, relaxing or exciting place or activity that brings you happiness. Exploring this place or activity in your mind in great detail can help induce a sense of calm.

> "When I began to panic or experience discomfort I'd close my eyes and concentrate on my own breathing until all I could hear was my breathing and heartbeat. Then I'd picture my toes and try to put them to sleep, and work my way up my legs, thighs, hips, arms, and hands until I felt very heavy. Once I achieved that heaviness, I'd try to picture a place I'd like to be and concentrate on the details. I pictured myself as sixteen-years-old, wearing a white gauzy dress, sitting with my dog on my favorite patchwork quilt in a forest glen with the rays of the sun coming through the trees. My long hair would be blowing in the breeze, and it felt good. After that, I would be calm."

Relaxation and imagery techniques are easy to learn but they take an initial investment of time, concentration and practice to master. There are a number of relaxation and imagery exercises online that can help you get started. Depending on the complexity of the relaxation technique and whether you're learning it alone or with guidance, it may require as much as one-to-two weeks of practice before you can use it effectively.

Experiment with several methods until you find one that's right for you and then stick with it. Since it can be hard to concentrate after chemotherapy or when you are uncomfortable, find an online audiotape that you can play to guide you through the exercise.

Hypnosis

Hypnosis is often used by therapists, combined with distraction and/or imagery, to help change the way you experience pain, time, sensations of heat, cold and touch, and a sense of connection to your body. Hypnosis may enable you to think about the painful area of your body as a separate, unconnected part, or shorten your perception of how long the painful experience lasts.

Some people have an easier time using hypnosis than others. Children, as a group, appear to be more hypnotizable than adults since they are less reality-bound and more willing to engage in fantasy. To locate a therapist in your area who is skilled in hypnosis, contact the department of behavioral medicine at a cancer center near you.

Physical Stimulation

Suffering is triggered by pain signals transmitted through the nervous system and spinal cord to the brain. One way to dull these pain signals is to provide a different, competing physical sensation.

Applying heat or cold to painful areas, for example, often masks pain signals and reduces suffering. Ice packs, however, should not be used for six months on skin that has been irradiated.

Massage can also provide a soothing sensation that competes with pain signals.

Some patients find exercise a potent pain reliever:

> "I developed a case of shingles (herpes zoster) after my transplant. I continued to have discomfort long after the sores had healed. I tried everything to control the pain

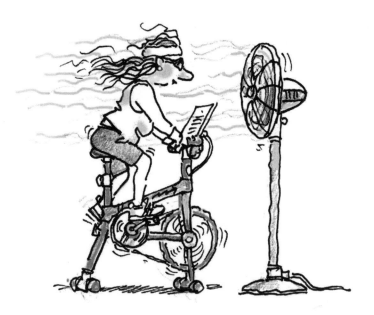

including acupuncture and pain pills. Nothing worked. Finally, I began to work out at the gym seven times a week. That turned out to be the best pain relief of all."

Learning to Use the Techniques

Learning non-drug pain control techniques before pain becomes intolerable is the key to using them successfully. Many hospitals with cancer programs offer classes that teach relaxation and imagery skills, or provide individual instruction and assistance.

While non-drug pain control techniques will usually not take the place of pain medications, they can give you a greater sense of control over your body and help make the healing process more tolerable.

Conclusion

After your transplant, don't hesitate to seek the help of a pain specialist if you feel your local physician is not taking your complaints of pain seriously or is unable to prescribe adequate pain medication. Most physicians have not received specialized training in pain control and some are more experienced than others in this rapidly evolving area of medicine.

Many universities and large hospitals now have special pain control programs with experts in both drug and non-drug pain control techniques who may be able to help you.

To watch helpful videos about managing pain, go to our website at:

bmtinfonet.org/video-manage-pain

Chapter Fourteen

FAMILY CAREGIVER

Pamper not only the patient, but the caregiver as well. The caregiver needs mail, home-cooked meals, a gift certificate to their favorite store, bath gel, something they would never get themselves (like music, a book, candy, colorful socks, a gourmet candy bar) — something to brighten their day and make them feel special. Even if you just send a $10 check with a note that says, 'Thought you could use a little extra something' — these things make a big difference. Long after the transplant, regardless of whether it's successful or not, memories of the experience will linger with the caregiver. Out of the blue, write or call. It's important that caregivers know you're still thinking of them.

Sarah, mother of a 22-month-old transplant patient

A blood stem cell transplant is not a procedure you can navigate alone.

Most transplant teams require patients to have a full-time caregiver to help during transplant and the recovery period, and will not allow the patient to go forward with a transplant unless a dedicated caregiver has been identified.

Typically, a close family member serves as the caregiver. If the patient does not have a close family member who can serve as a caregiver, he or she may need to reach out to extended family members or friends for help, or hire a temporary caregiver. Some patients assemble a team of caregivers.

While the patient is undergoing treatment, he or she will likely be too ill and weak to manage medical and household affairs without help for several weeks or months. A full-time family caregiver can help ensure that the patient gets prompt medical attention and that the house is a safe environment.

While the patient is in the hospital, the family caregiver will be responsible for:

- telling the medical team about any changes in the patient's condition
- providing the patient with emotional support
- advocating for the patient and helping with decision-making
- communicating with family and friends

After the patient is discharged from the hospital, the caregiver will assume additional duties including:

- transporting the patient to the outpatient clinic daily or weekly
- keeping track of medical appointments
- making sure the patient takes his or her medications according to schedule
- taking care of dressings and the central venous catheter
- reporting changes in the patient's condition to the medical team
- watching for signs of infection and other complications
- encouraging the patient to eat
- in some cases, giving the patient intravenous medications
- cleaning and cooking according to the guidelines provided by the transplant team
- protecting the patient from sources of infection, such as visitors with colds or those who have been around sick people
- helping the patient move around safely

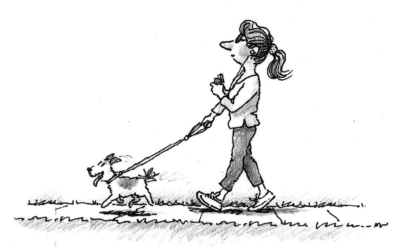

Taking Time to Recharge

As everyone's attention focuses on saving the patient's life, the needs of one of the patient's most important partners — the family member or friend who is the primary caregiver — are often underestimated.

In order to provide the best possible care for the patient, caregivers need to take time off to recharge. There are many things that can be done to relieve the stress of caregiving, get a clear head and find a little bit of perspective. Whether you choose to go for a walk, take in a movie, visit with friends, or just take a nap, taking time for yourself is essential, say former caregivers.

> "Even though you may not want to or think you need to, getting away from the caregiving world for even half an hour is important. One person, even a workaholic, can't handle this situation alone."

"You're going to feel tired, frustrated, even annoyed at your loved one sometimes, and that's OK. It's a very stressful time for everyone and you are only human. Even though you love the person going through the transplant, there will be days when you are just plain tired of the hospital, the disease and the treatment. Try to take some time for yourself. Go for a walk outside. Get away from the hospital if just for a few minutes. Write in a journal, read a book, work on a project (I put photos in an album). You are not being selfish. You have to take time for yourself in order to really help your loved one."

The need to take time for yourself doesn't end when the transplant is over, and the patient returns home. At home, you will have to assume many tasks that were handled by nurses in the hospital or clinic. It is critical to pace yourself because you may be giving care intensively for a long time.

"When my wife came home from the hospital, caring for her was even harder than it was while she was hospitalized. I no longer had nurses and doctors on hand to monitor her, and I had to be constantly vigilant to detect problems. That was a lot of stress.

During times when the patient is not in danger, try to take a few hours away for yourself. You will be under a lot of stress for the long-haul, and you need to get some relief."

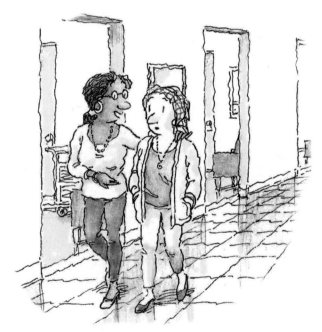

Some caregivers find that classes on how to care for chronically ill patients, offered at some hospitals or health agencies, help ease the strain.

"The transplant center instructed me on things specific to transplant patients, like how to take care of the catheter. But courses for caregivers of chronically ill patients, offered at our local hospital, were also helpful. They taught the basics of caring for chronically ill patients — like how to help them without disrupting the household, how to help them walk without injuring yourself, etc. It was basic information that would be covered in a nursing assistance course."

Taking Care of Physical Well-Being

A caregiver is only effective if he or she is in good physical condition. Constantly overdoing it can backfire. Eat well balanced meals, exercise and sleep when you can. You need to stay well in order to take proper care of the patient.

"Learn, develop and practice good self-care skills prior to the transplant. Once the transplant begins, your primary attention will be on the patient, and you'll have little time or energy left to learn these skills."

"I knew from the start I was in for a long haul and had to take care of myself. I set 11 p.m. as my curfew and let my wife know I had to leave the hospital then so I could sleep and come back in the morning refreshed. I pretty much stuck to that except for those nights when things weren't going well. When I stayed overnight at the hospital, I really paid for it for the next two to three days."

Managing Feelings

One of the complexities of being a caregiver is that it's not neutral—caregivers are taking care of patients about whom they care deeply. People who have done it stress the importance of having a forum for processing feelings and fears apart from the patient. Don't count on the patient to understand your emotional needs. Lean on others for support.

"Don't get so caught up worrying about everyone else that you don't deal with your own feelings and fears. Find a counselor or someone who understands what you are going

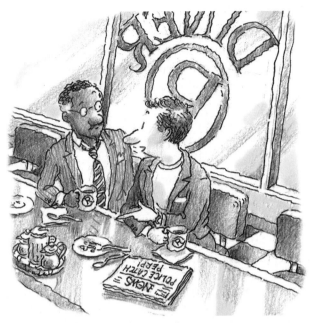

through and talk your feelings out. Allow yourself to cry. I say this because I didn't do this, and after several months of anxiety, I started having physical symptoms. If you don't deal with your feelings, they will deal with you."

The importance of emotional support for caregivers cannot be emphasized too much. Find someone who is a good listener, who will let you talk about your feelings. Some caregivers find a special friend or small circle of friends works well. Others find the families of other transplant patients most helpful. Professional counseling or talks with clergy help many caregivers deal with the experience.

"It helps to have your own network of friends whose number one concern is how you are doing. The caregiver is so busy worrying about what the patient needs, you often don't recognize your own feelings. I had a few family members and friends who would contact me periodically to see how I was doing. I kept a diary and would send it to them, and they'd call or write in response. Their calls made me sit down and think about how I was really feeling."

"I frequently talked with other families on the transplant unit — they were in as much pain as I was and understood what I was going through. We all helped each other other. We were one big family."

"Seek counseling or the help of a spiritual advisor before the transplant begins. This experience changed my belief system on a very deep level and in ways I could not have predicted. I was grateful to have an already established channel for expressing and discussing these changes."

BMT InfoNet's Caring Connections Program can link you with other caregivers who have been through a similar experience. Go to bmtinfonet.org/caring-connection or phone 888-597-7674.

Accepting Help

Planning for the long haul includes inviting and accepting help from others. Many people assume that the transplant is simply their own problem to manage. Yet taking care of a very sick patient and managing the usual household and work chores is more than most people can handle.

Extended family members and friends often truly want to help, but don't know what would be most appreciated. Figure out what people are good at and give them jobs that suit their temperament and skills.

- If someone enjoys physical activity, let that friend cut the grass or shovel snow.
- Good cooks can prepare meals.
- A friend can run to the grocery store or pharmacy to pick up needed items.
- Parents of your children's friends can help drive your children to school and after-school activities.

Develop a strong network of support before the transplant. This will free you up to focus on the patient's needs.

"One of the hardest things for both of us to learn was to let other people help us. We weren't used to having other people do things for us. We always assumed there would have to be a payback.

But people would take the kids shopping for school clothes, take them to the show, etc. and refuse money when I offered it to them. Finally we had to accept the fact that we could never repay everyone for their kindness. There were too many people helping us for that. It made a big change in our lives to realize how many friends we really had."

You may want to designate one person to coordinate volunteers. Online programs like MealTrain.com or LotsofHelpingHands.org are useful tools to schedule meals and other services for your family.

Being the Patient's Advocate

Part of being the patient's caregiver is being his or her advocate. Caregivers know information about the patient that doctors and nurses may not have. You may know, for example, how best to get your child to do unpleasant tasks. If you are caring for an adult patient, you may know that he or she will be reluctant to ask for pain relief before the pain is severe and more difficult to control.

Although the transplant team works hard to provide the best care for patients, they may not always pick up patient distress signals as easily as a caregiver who knows the patient well. It comforts patients to know that their caregiver is looking out for their well-being only, and is not distracted by the needs of other patients.

"I saw my job as a gatekeeper — keeping track of details, asking questions, being an advocate for my wife with the medical staff and taking care of her emotional and physical needs. I was present at all the medical consultations and made sure I paid attention to details like whether she was receiving proper medicines. When visitors came I managed them, depending on whether or not my wife wanted to see them."

Getting Information

Although getting information on a daily basis from the patient's doctor is important, it's sometimes hard to accomplish. Find out when the doctors make their rounds each day so you can be there to ask questions. If you are unable to be present when the doctor visits, find out when you can contact him or her by phone or visit in person.

> "I made a point of becoming very well informed about the transplant process. I felt strongly that I was an advocate for my husband, and in order to be taken seriously and to get the best care for him, I had to be knowledgeable. At the same time, I worked hard to ignore statistics. They're useful for scientists, but not patients. A person cannot be 20% alive and 80% dead, so it's pointless to get hung up on the numbers."

One family who had multiple caregivers left a journal with the patient. All caregivers wrote in it daily about the patient's medical care, other important details, and feelings. Some people even tape recorded or videotaped meetings with doctors to help them keep track of important information.

> "Keep a diary and carry it with you. Write down everything in it — doctors' instructions, names, phone numbers, maps, etc. One day starts to blend into the next and it becomes impossible to remember everything without taking notes."

Be prepared for the fact that the physicians rotate off duty each month. Find out when doctors rotate so you can debrief the doctor who is leaving, get some information about the doctor who is about to assume your loved one's care, and prepare the patient for the change.

Flexibility and Patience: Essential Components

As it is with many things in life, each transplant evolves in its own way. There is no way to predict how someone's course will unfold. You'll need to be prepared for ups and downs during the patient's treatment and recovery. Complications can occur, and recovery sometimes takes longer than expected.

After the patient returns home, there can be setbacks. It's common for transplant patients to develop infections and other complications that may require them to be admitted to the hospital.

"Plan all you can, but expect the unexpected. Plan to be more tired than you can possibly imagine. Take things one day at a time or, if necessary, one hour at a time and hang in there."

"I tried to say the serenity prayer every day. God, grant me the serenity to accept things I cannot change, courage to change the things I can, and the wisdom to know the difference."

Keeping a Sense of Humor

Many caregivers say that maintaining a sense of humor, despite the difficulties, helped them and the patient cope.

"Through all the tears, we managed to find a lot of humor — which kept us all sane. Sometimes things that seem so traumatic at the time can really strike you funny in retrospect.

For example, when my sister was having her chemotherapy, the nurses suggested she shave off her hair, rather than let it fall out. My dad wanted to take pictures of it, and we really argued with him about it — it was so upsetting at the time. But a few days later, when we looked at the pictures, we all had a good laugh. We couldn't believe we'd been fighting over hair, when there were so many bigger issues at stake."

"I would rent funny movies or read funny books to my wife. I also found it helpful to share humorous moments with visitors and friends. The transplant was very scary for our friends. My wife and I were in deep denial as we went through it, but our friends understood the severity of the situation. It made it easier for them to call or visit if we could share some humorous moments with them."

> "Pray, cry and talk when you need to, but also keep a positive attitude. During my husband's recovery, we played a lot of cards, talked about all the fun we'd had, and all the fun we were going to have once he was well."

Relaying Information to Others

One task many caregivers find draining is keeping family and friends informed about the patient's progress. Relying on friends to help with this task eases the burden. So does relying on technology.

Consider setting up a communication network in advance with family, co-workers and friends.

> "It was really draining to get information to all the people who cared. After working all day and being at the hospital, it takes all your energy just to exist some days. My wife and I shared details with four or five close friends who we knew would be a great source of support. For the rest, I recorded a more general message each day on our voice mail."

> "I sent a summary of the week's events to family and friends each Saturday night. I began writing in a journal the day my wife went into the hospital. I spent a half hour to one hour each day recording events and our feelings. Initially I did it so my wife would have a record of what happened to her. But it became the way I organized my thoughts, sorted out feelings, and communicated with loved ones. I've continued journaling even to this day."

CaringBridge.org is an excellent way to keep family and friends up-to-date about the patient's progress and allow friends and family to post messages and well-wishes for the patient.

Know Your Role

Caring for an adult who is undergoing a stem cell transplant is emotionally difficult and physically exhausting. Not only do you have to juggle the needs of the patient, your own needs, and those of your family members, but you must do it without help from the person with whom you normally share these responsibilities — the patient.

> "I think it's tougher for the caregiver than the patient. All of the patient's energies are focused on getting well, but you also have your normal day-to-day stuff like work, children, bills and other family members to deal with. It's a lot of stress."

To complicate matters, you and the patient may have different ideas about the caregiver's role. You may feel you have to become a medical expert to properly care for the patient when, in reality, what the patient may want most is emotional support.

> "Find out what the patient expects of you. My husband just wanted me there, not to entertain him, but for companionship, and to give support and comfort during the long recovery process."

> "It helps to follow the cues of the patient. Do as little or as much as he wants you to do. Help the patient maintain his dignity by letting him take the lead."

Walking the thin line between being an understanding caregiver, and wanting the patient to take a more active role in his or her recovery can be difficult. Sometimes caregivers feel that the patient should be making more progress, but don't know how hard to push the issue.

> "Be patient, but also feel your way into becoming more assertive with the patient. I always felt I shouldn't say certain things to my husband, but then I started feeling depressed and isolated. I waited too long to tell him simple things, like he had enough strength to take out the garbage. He became extremely depressed and dependent on me. That was very hard, but eventually we worked things out."

> "Getting the patient to bathe, eat, exercise and take medications is not always easy. Sometimes you have to be stern with instructions. Learn to be patient, but kindly persistent. A good caregiver is not a softy."

Changing Relationships

Being the caregiver for an adult, particularly a spouse, who is recovering from a transplant can dramatically alter your relationship — at least for a time.

The physical and emotional trauma experienced by both you and the patient may sometimes be expressed as anger, irritability or

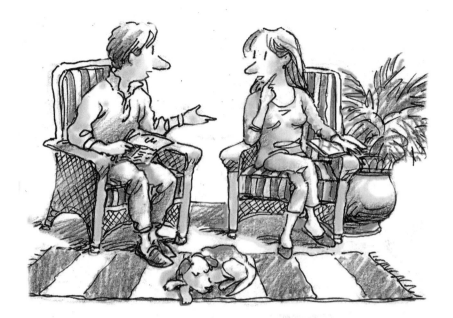

depression. In most cases, the problems resolve over time and some eventually share a closer relationship with their spouse. For others, the changes remain for a long time.

> "I had to take over all of his responsibilities —paying bills, yard work, etc. Instead of being an equal partner, it was like having another child to worry about. I felt like I'd lost the man I married and just wanted him back."

> "We seem to have permanently traded roles. He used to be the more relaxed, practical, conscientious partner. Now I have to constantly remind him not to get upset over little things and to be more positive."

> "The changes we've noticed are for the better. We made it through one of the most difficult things a couple can go through. It has changed our perspective and led us to make a number of positive changes in our lives. Which is not to say that we don't still fight about nothing from time to time, but rather that our fighting is half-hearted, as though we know it's nothing."

Helping Children Cope

Children of transplant patients share in the trauma of their parent's illness and treatment. Depending on their age, they may express their fears in a number of different ways.

- Some become depressed.

- Others have behavioral problems, difficulties at school, or begin to regress.

- Still others may worry that they caused or will catch the disease.

For most children, just being separated from their parent for a long period of time is very distressing. Being open and honest with children about the parent's disease and treatment, and allowing them to express their questions and concerns is essential to helping them cope with the experience.

> "Our three children, ages two, seven, and eleven, had all kinds of problems. The stress of knowing their mother might not live was overwhelming. I tried to help them by talking with them, over and over again, about my wife's illness. I made sure they understood that there are no stupid questions or feelings."

> "My 13-year-old son became very depressed while his father was undergoing a transplant out of town. In addition to getting him some professional help, I sent him to visit his father over Spring break. It helped him to see his father alive and progressing."

> "A big concern expressed by our six-year-old daughter was that her mom was going to be bald. We took control of the situation by first taking her to the hospital several times before the transplant to see other people and children who were bald. We then made it a 'family outing' with friends and a movie camera when my wife went to the hairdresser and had her hair buzzed army-style. Our daughter accepted the baldness well and even asked to take her mom to school for 'show and tell'. She was very proud of her bald mom, and my wife went with no reservations."

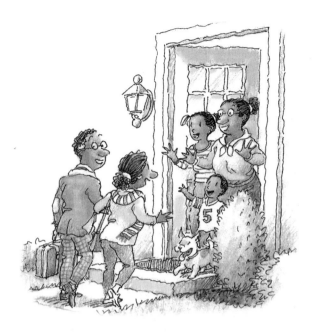

Coming Home

Everyone looks forward to leaving the hospital or ending the daily visits to the outpatient clinic. Many, however, are unprepared for the fact that for the first months, life at home will not be normal.

In many ways, caring for a transplant patient at home is more difficult than assisting with his or her care while in the hospital or outpatient clinic.

- Medications must be administered.
- Catheters must be carefully cleaned.
- Special diets may have to be followed.
- Infection precautions must be adhered to.

All this must be done at home without the help of a readily available nursing staff.

The early weeks and months are often a confusing and stressful time for families. This is a time when many caregivers experience burn-out. Your loved one has survived the rigors of the treatment and you should be happy, but the difficulties are far from over.

There are frequent clinic visits, sometimes a hospitalization, and ongoing caregiving responsibilities. Support systems may begin to fall apart as family and friends mistakenly think that life is now back to normal.

> "Picking up the pieces is not easy. For months I felt like I was on autopilot. I forgot how to sleep and constantly felt like I was dragging. There didn't seem to be enough hours in the day or energy in me to take care of everyone's needs. After ten months I wondered, 'When will this be over?'"

It's good to let friends and family members know how they can help. Although some may not be as understanding as you'd like, others will be glad for the opportunity to help and be thankful that you are explicit about what you need.

Conclusion

Happily, most people who survive a stem cell transplant report that it was worth the difficulties. Caregivers survive, too, although probably changed from the people they were before the experience.

> "Some good came out of this experience, aside from the fact that my daughter is alive. It helped everyone think about what is important in life."

Perhaps this three-and-a-half-year-old survivor said it best to his mom about the importance of caregivers:

> "On the first anniversary of his transplant, I told him it was time to visit the clinic again and he asked, 'Why?' I said, 'Everyone who took care of you wants to see you and besides, we should thank the doctors for making you better.' He looked at me and said, 'No, mommy, you made me better.'"

To learn more, go to our website at:

bmtinfonet.org/role-of-caregiver

Chapter Fifteen
PLANNING FOR SURVIVORSHIP

"The transition from being sick to being healthy can be really difficult. There is a tension that exists because you're going back to the life you once knew, but you may not feel like the same person you were before. So, you have to really practice living in the present moment so that your mind doesn't get the best of you."

Melanie, eight-year transplant survivor

As a transplant survivor, you have been through an extraordinary experience. As you move forward with your life, you may find yourself feeling different — different from the people around you and different than your former self.

Survivorship may mean a new appreciation of life, new interests or new priorities. It also may mean getting used to side effects and learning to function despite them. Although many of these side effects will resolve by the end of the first year after transplant, some survivors must adjust to side effects long-term.

Transplant survivors find joy in the fact that they have been given a new lease on life. However, protecting your health long-term requires a good understanding of the treatment you've undergone and your risk for developing complications later on. It also requires access to healthcare providers who are knowledgeable about transplantation and its late effects, and can monitor you for long-term complications.

Survivorship Care Plan

Although some patients can return to their transplant center for long-term follow-up care, many cannot. Most community primary care physicians and oncologists have received little or no training in the care of transplant survivors. Thus, you will need a good long-term follow-up plan prepared by your transplant team that outlines your medical history, treatments you received and potential long-term issues that may arise so that your local doctors can provide you with the best care possible. This is sometimes called a Survivorship Care Plan.

The symptoms of some complications can resemble other disorders local doctors often see. Younger transplant survivors can also have effects such as high cholesterol or diabetes that doctors do not expect to see until people are older. Therefore they are not looking for these complications. Without knowledge of your medical background, your local doctor may miss checking for some problems or may direct you to specialists or prescribe tests that will miss the actual problem.

YOU are an important partner in protecting your health long-term. The more informed you are about your treatment history and risk for long-term complications, the better equipped you will be to advocate for appropriate long-term care. If you have a Survivorship Care Plan, you can discuss it with your doctor and know that your health needs are being watched.

What Should Be In the Plan?

When you no longer require care at the transplant center, ask your transplant team to prepare a long-term plan for follow-up care. Ideally, your long-term follow-up plan should include the following information:

- the date, dosage and type of chemotherapy you received, including any you received prior to being referred to the transplant center, especially if you received a type of medication called an anthracycline such as doxorubicin (Adriamycin®)
- the date, type and site of any radiation you received including any you received prior to being referred to the transplant center

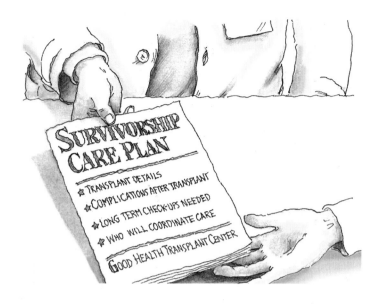

- other medications you received while being treated for your disease that have potential long-term health effects such as steroids
- any serious infections you developed and how they were treated
- other major complications that could have long-term effects
- whether you developed graft-versus-host disease, how it was treated and how long it was treated
- if you relapsed after transplant, how it was treated
- potential late effects for each therapy you received including mental health effects and cognitive effects
- a list of your medications and allergies
- a list of your vaccinations
- copies of test results to share with your local doctors
- a list of tests and clinical evaluations that should be done periodically to detect possible problems and their frequency
- whom your doctor should contact for questions and instructions

Make several copies of your long-term follow-up plan and be sure to give it to each of your doctors that you see regularly, including dentists. Because you have a complicated medical history, you will need to take responsibility for making sure that all of your doctors know about any medical issues that can arise after transplant.

It is important to have a primary care provider that you trust. Discuss with that doctor, physician assistant or nurse practitioner if he or she is available to coordinate your care so that all the members of your healthcare team are up-to-date on your health history. This will not only help to make sure you get the tests and clinical exams you need but also make sure you are not getting duplicated tests or more than you need.

Be sure that your transplant team knows the names and contact information for all doctors who are currently caring for you. Update that information annually, particularly if you are changing doctors.

Long-Term Follow-Up Care and Tests

Guidelines for long-term follow-up care have been developed by the Center for International Blood and Marrow Transplant Research (CIBMTR), a leading scientific organization that conducts research on blood stem cell transplantation, and six other international medical societies.

The guidelines are written in lay language for patients, and include a summary sheet of tests and periodic exams that you need which should be given to each of your doctors. A link to the guidelines can be found on BMT InfoNet's website at bmtinfonet.org/long-term-health-guidelines.

The Children's Oncology Group has similar guidelines for children who have undergone cancer therapy. These guidelines take into account the effect various chemotherapy drugs and radiation may have on growing children and, thus, include a number of tests and exams not needed by adults. You can find a link to these guidelines at survivorshipguidelines.org.

Steps you and your local doctors can take to protect your health after transplant include:

- redo your childhood vaccinations using the plan advised by your transplant team, usually six-to-twelve months after transplant

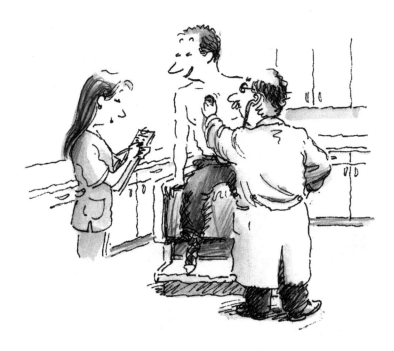

- check with your transplant team about an additional vaccination plan for you since these recommendations can change
- check with your transplant team whether your annual flu vaccine should be with an inactivated vaccine
- tests to evaluate your risk of infection
- pulmonary function tests to evaluate your lungs, especially if lung abnormalities are present after transplant
- an ophthalmology exam to check your vision and determine whether you are forming cataracts
- annual dental exam to check your teeth and mouth for cavities, dry mouth, gum disease and oral cancer
- annual thyroid function tests
- tests to check your kidney and liver function
- checking sex hormone levels
- annual cholesterol and other tests to check your heart and blood vessel function

- annual glucose test for diabetes
- bone density tests to check for osteoporosis, if you are at risk

If the survivor is a child, additional testing will be required to monitor growth, sexual development, learning ability and early onset of heart problems.

Emotional Well-Being

Emotional distress is common among transplant survivors, at least for a while. It is a significant problem for caregivers as well.

Stress can be caused by a number of factors:

- fear of relapse
- living with uncertainties about the future
- changes in body image
- a slow rate of recovery
- medical setbacks
- being socially isolated
- financial burdens
- not feeling that people really understand what you and your family are going through

Some survivors find that support groups, online chat rooms or ongoing relationships with other survivors provide the best emotional support.

> "They had a reunion at my transplant center last year and a big patient meeting was held. The first thing you know, someone raised her hand and said, 'Has anyone ever experienced such and such problem?' Well, we were off and running. Somebody else said, 'Do you have memory problems?' I described it differently and other people said, 'Yeah, yeah, that's it.' The meeting was a huge success and we all came out grinning because for the first time we were able to get these issues out on the table and get some information about them."

Although face-to-face support groups for transplant survivors are rare, there are online support groups and telephone support programs that many survivors find helpful.

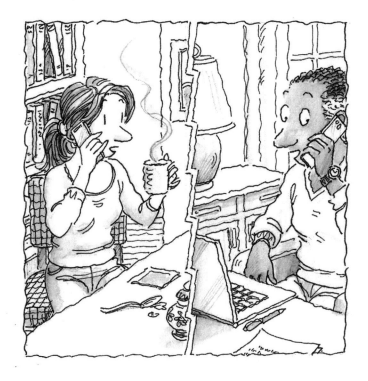

BMT InfoNet offers a Caring Connections Program to link patients and family members who need emotional support with others who understand what they are going through. You can request a Caring Connection at bmtinfonet.org/caring-connection or by phoning 888-597-7674.

There are many Facebook and other online groups where transplant recipients can connect. You can "like" BMT InfoNet's Bone Marrow and Stem Cell Transplant Club on Facebook, or join our closed Facebook group for survivors BMT InfoNet Celebrating a 2nd Chance at Life.

The services of a psychiatrist, psychologist, social worker or other counselor help some survivors get back a sense of well-being.

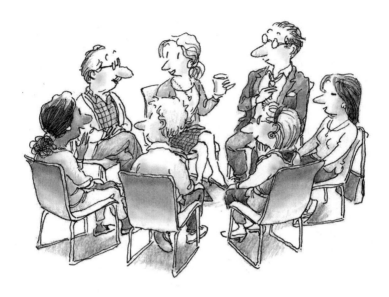

"Fifteen months later when I ended the counseling sessions, I thanked the psychiatrist and told him, 'My transplant doctor gave me back my life, but you put the quality back in my life.'"

Some survivors experience survivor guilt. It may happen when another transplant patient they know relapses or does not survive the transplant. Support groups, counseling and clergy can be good resources to help manage these feelings.

Fear of relapse, along with uncertainty about what could go wrong, is a major stress for many people, particularly during the early years after transplant. It may take a long time before you feel comfortable making long-term plans or spending a day without thinking about your disease or treatment.

Worries about relapse are completely normal, especially before you have check-ups or if you have a new health problem. If this fear or worry is interfering with your ability to enjoy life, ask for a referral to a therapist or counselor who has experience helping people who have gone through treatment for a life-threatening illness.

Changing Relationships with Family Members

Marriages often change after transplant. Some couples report that their relationship is the same or better than before the transplant. For others the opposite is true.

> "Without a doubt, going through the transplant strengthened our marital relationship. We threw out all the trash that had accumulated over the years and got our priorities straight."

> "After my transplant, I changed in ways that my wife couldn't understand. I wanted to go a million miles an hour and experience everything. Activities and friends that were now very important to me seemed trivial to her. Our marriage finally ended in divorce last Fall."

> "The whole experience frightened my husband to no end. You don't realize how hard it is on the spouse until it's all over. He doesn't want to talk about it, think about it or hear about it. I couldn't even get him to congratulate me on my transplant anniversary. Don't get me wrong, he's a great guy and we love each other very much. But it would be nice to be able to talk with him about the experience sometimes."

Relationships with children can also change after transplant.

> "The transplant was very hard on my daughters who were sixteen, thirteen and two at the time. They were terrified of losing their mother, and each of them showed their stress in a different way. The oldest felt responsible for the younger two if I died, and that was a big burden for someone her age. Even after I came home, my middle one was afraid that I would be sick again, and didn't know how to talk about her fears. The little one literally clung to me for two years.

> Working through these problems was a long ordeal, but they've all grown to be very mature, responsible kids. I'm very proud of them and they're proud of me."

A family therapist may be able to help you work through strained relationships and enable each party to understand the other's perspective. Keeping the lines of communication open is key.

The Bottom Line

It may take a while before the constant worrying about your health is over for both you and your loved ones. While physical well-being is important, strong family relationships, friendships, inner spirituality and helping others are also important factors that make for a good quality of life. Many survivors feel the transplant experience helped them get their priorities straight and prompted them to live each day to the fullest, rather than put off the important things for the future.

When struggling with setbacks or feeling like things will never be normal, you may find it helpful to review or even write down five things in your life today that you are grateful for. It doesn't make the problems go away, but it can help to put things into better balance.

Some transplant survivors say the experience taught them a lot about what their bodies and minds are capable of doing. Prior to the transplant, everyone is frightened of potential physical complications and pain, and most survivors experience emotional ups and downs for many months following the transplant. Yet, they find ways to cope with these problems and enjoy their second chance at life.

> "It took almost two years for me to adjust and reshape my life. It required counseling, support group meetings, constant family support, the loyalty and help from friends and a renewed faith in God. I am now a reasonably happy and content survivor. I've gained peace of mind and peace of soul. I'm finally getting a glimpse of who I really am, and I like what I'm seeing. I still have lingering complications, but if I never feel any better physically than I do right now, I'll still count my blessings. The transplant was, indeed, a traumatic experience, but it gave me the only chance I had to live, and I'm glad that I took it."

For more on long-term health guidelines, go to

bmtinfonet.org/long-term-health-guidelines

Chapter Sixteen
LATE EFFECTS IN ADULTS AND CHILDREN

The bone marrow transplant affected my life in every way. I am thankful to wake up each morning. I have learned compassion and empathy for those unable to be 'normal'. I have learned how much it means when others are kind. I have learned the value of a family in my life. I have had a paper on my refrigerator for the last five years that reads, 'My goal is to live forever, so far, so good.' The seasons change on our Iowa farm, the crops and animals grow. I, too, hope to keep changing and growing.

Kathleen, 22-year survivor of two transplants

Some of the complications associated with stem cell transplantation are not apparent until several months, or even years after treatment. Most of them resolve with time, but others may be permanent and need attention long-term. Still others may not appear until 10 or 20 years after transplant.

Late effects of transplant may include:

- chronic graft-versus-host disease (cGVHD)
- heart and blood vessel problems
- metabolic problems (diabetes, thyroid, other hormones)
- secondary cancers
- infection

- attention and memory problems
- chronic fatigue and sleep issues
- vision problems
- bone loss
- neuropathy (numbness and tingling in hands and feet)
- kidney or lung issues
- sexual difficulties
- infertility

No one experiences all of these complications. Your risk for developing problems after transplant will depend on:

- your disease
- the amount and type of chemotherapy and radiation you had
- your age
- prior treatment history

Many complications that affect your quality of life can be prevented with proper screening and prompt treatment.

Chronic Graft-versus-Host Disease (cGVHD)

Chronic graft-versus-host disease (cGVHD) is a complication that affects approximately 50 percent of patients who undergo an allogeneic transplant.

Chronic GVHD typically develops three or more months after transplant, but it can begin earlier as well. Most cases of cGVHD are mild or moderate, but serious – even life-threatening – cGVHD can occur as well.

(For a detailed description of chronic GVHD, the organs it affects and treatment options go to Chapter Ten, Graft-versus-Host Disease.)

Heart and Blood Vessel Problems

The incidence of coronary artery disease and cardiomyopathy (heart muscle disease that weakens the heart) is three time higher among transplant recipients than the general population. Risk factors include:

- anthracycline chemotherapies such as doxorubicin (Adriamycin®)
- radiation to the chest (not total body irradiation)
- other chemotherapies such as cyclophosphamide (Cytoxan®) and melphalan
- hormonal changes
- inactivity and muscle loss

To protect your heart:

- have regular check-ups for blood pressure, diabetes and cholesterol
- exercise regularly, including muscle building exercises
- do not smoke
- eat a low-fat diet to maintain a healthy weight

High blood pressure, triglycerides or cholesterol often occur as people age. However, after transplant they can happen even in young adults. You want to pay attention to these because, if they are not treated effectively they can cause early heart attacks or strokes.

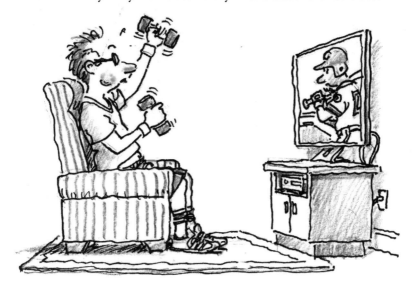

It is important that your doctors test you for these problems at your annual physical exam. But it is also important that they follow-up to make sure your treatment is working. It is common for transplant survivors to be under-treated when these problems are diagnosed. It is important for you to stay on top of your care and follow-up with your doctor.

Another less common but difficult problem is a disease of the heart muscles called cardiomyopathy. This problem sometimes happens if you are treated with a type of chemotherapy called an anthracycline, such as doxorubicin. It can also happen if your heart is exposed to high-dose radiation therapy.

Your doctor should look at the dosage of the anthracyclines or radiation therapy you received to assess your risk of cardiomyopathy. Tests for cardiomyopathy may include an echocardiogram and/or an MRI of the heart. Although cardiomyopathy cannot be fixed, it is helpful to know whether it is a problem so your doctor can monitor the situation and create an appropriate treatment plan for you.

Metabolic (Hormone) Problems

When we think about hormones, we usually think about male and female hormones such as testosterone or estrogen. These can affect sexual responses, mood and energy. But there are other hormones that are every bit as important that can be impacted by transplant.

Thyroid problems such as hypothyroidism (a low level of the thyroid hormone) are common after transplant. These problems are treatable so you should have your
thyroid monitored every year.

Another much less common complication after transplant is when the adrenal glands produce less cortisol than you need. This 'adrenal insufficiency' can cause fatigue, weakness and other problems. Although this problem is less common, you should be tested for it when you have your annual physical exam and blood tests.

A common problem after allogeneic transplant is elevated glucose levels or 'insulin resistance.' This can lead to diabetes which often occurs together with high cholesterol. The combination can be particularly concerning after transplant since over time it can lead to heart attacks or strokes.

On the positive side, diabetes can be treated with medication along with lifestyle changes that also make you feel good. You will want to have a fasting glucose test every year.

If you have one or more of these complications after transplant, your doctor may refer you to an endocrinologist to monitor and treat your hormone problem.

Attention and Memory Problems

For many patients, a surprising side effect of transplant is a change in the way they process information. These changes are called cognitive changes and can be very frustrating for both the survivor and family caregiver.

In some patients cognitive changes are very subtle. In others they are more severe.

You may experience:

- memory lapses
- trouble concentrating
- difficulty multitasking
- problems with organization
- difficulty remembering words during a conversation

These problems usually diminish or completely resolve over time, but some patients continue to experience cognitive issues long-term.

Consult a neurologist if the problem persists. There are a variety of strategies you can use to function well despite the changes. Go to bmtinfonet.org/cognitive for tips on how to manage cognitive problems.

Chronic Fatigue

Chronic fatigue is a common complaint following transplant. It can interfere with mood, physical activity, job performance and sleep. Unlike the fatigue we experience in everyday life, rest does not always relieve it.

Fatigue can be caused by a number of factors including:

- anemia
- depression
- pain
- sleep disorders
- electrolyte disturbances
- infection
- poorly functioning immune system
- thyroid disorder
- adrenal insufficiency
- malnutrition
- dehydration
- lack of exercise which leads to deconditioning
- stress
- medications that act on the brain and spinal cord
- inflammatory agents such as IL-6, cytokines and interferons

Survivors who experience fatigue after transplant often complain about decreased energy, a generalized weakness and/or decreased motivation. Fatigue can cause sadness, frustration and irritability. It can make it difficult to perform daily tasks and affect memory.

Be sure to report chronic fatigue to your healthcare team. There are a number of tests that can be performed to check for possible causes like anemia, thyroid problems or adrenal insufficiency which can be easy to treat.

Drinking sufficient liquids and consuming enough carbohydrates and protein are important tools in managing fatigue. Your transplant team can refer you to a nutritionist who can help develop a plan tailored to your needs.

Conserve your energy for the times of the day that you need it most.

- Plan to do necessary activities at the time of day when you have the most energy.
- Pace yourself, avoid rushing and delegate responsibilities when possible.
- Gradually increase exercise to build muscle and overcome fatigue.

Exercise and physical activity can improve symptoms of fatigue. Even five-to-ten minutes of exercise several times daily can help. Consider enrolling in an exercise class at a gym or local yoga studio to maintain a schedule of physical exercise. Ask a physical therapist to recommend exercises or a gym that will understand and adapt to your needs as a transplant survivor.

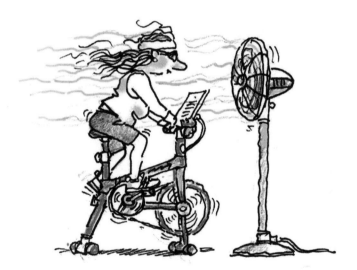

A number of medications can also provide short-term relief from fatigue such as Provigil®, Neuvigil®, Ritalin® and Adderal®. Cognitive behavioral therapy can also help manage fatigue.

Sometimes fatigue can affect you mentally. If you find that you concentrate well for an hour or two and then it seems like your brain doesn't focus, it may be caused by mental fatigue. Rather than trying to push through and becoming frustrated, try taking a break and giving your body and brain some down time to recover. You may find it easier to get back on track after a break.

If fatigue interferes with your ability to work, consider talking with your employer about alternate ways to manage your workload. Set realistic goals, perhaps shorten hours or request a disability leave of absence. Don't be embarrassed to ask for help. This is one of the most common problems after transplant.

TriageCancer.org/employment has information about employment rights that you may find helpful. CancerandCareers.org is another excellent resource for cancer survivors who need help with employment issues.

Learn more about managing chronic fatigue at bmtinfonet.org/fatigue-and-sleep.

Difficulty Sleeping

Sleep problems are common among transplant survivors, as well as family caregivers, and can persist for years. Insufficient sleep over a long period of time can create serious health problems such as heart disease, diabetes and obesity.

Poor sleep can also contribute to:

- headaches
- daytime fatigue
- depression
- anxiety
- substance abuse
- attention, concentration and memory problems
- irritability

Doctors often prescribe sleep medication for insomnia. However, you may also be able to achieve a good night's rest without medication using cognitive behavioral therapy designed specifically for insomnia (CBT-I). In fact, the American College of Physicians recommends that all adult patients receive cognitive-behavioral therapy for insomnia as the initial treatment, rather than medication.

Cognitive behavioral therapy for insomnia helps patients understand their sleep, and change the thoughts and behaviors that interfere with sleep. In six-to-eight sessions over a few months, a therapist who specializes in CBT-I helps you:

- track and understand your current sleep behavior
- identify behaviors that interfere with sleep
- adopt habits that promote a good night's rest
- become aware of negative thoughts about sleep that worsen sleep problems

Sleep-promoting habits that a therapist might help you develop include:

- establishing a regular sleep schedule
- waking up at the same time each day, including weekends
- using your bed only for sleep and sex
- getting out of bed at night, rather than lying awake, if you are having trouble falling asleep
- prior to bedtime, making a list of things you need to do the next day, so you don't stay awake worrying if you will remember them

You can find a trained sleep therapist through the Society for Behavioral Sleep Medicine at behavioralsleep.org or by phoning 859-312-8880. If none exists in your area, try these print resources:

- Overcoming Insomnia, by Jack D. Edinger and Colleen E. Carney
- The Insomnia Workbook, by Stephanie A. Silberman, PhD, DABSM
- Say Good Night to Insomnia, by Gregg D. Jacobs, PhD

There are also online cognitive behavioral therapy programs for people with sleep issues such as Sleepio.com that may be helpful.

If you have been taking sleep medication since your transplant, or for a long-time, do not just stop your medication 'cold turkey.' You can develop side effects that can be very uncomfortable and can cause a lot of suffering. Talk with your doctor about a plan to gradually reduce your medication.

For more about managing sleep problems go to bmtinfonet.org/video-manage-sleep.

Vision Problems

Cataracts are a common side effect of transplant. If you develop a cataract, it can be surgically removed in an outpatient setting.

If you had total body irradiation, you may experience dry eyes after transplant. The problem can usually be managed with artificial tears or ointments.

Chronic graft-versus-host disease can cause dry eyes and vision problems. (See Chapter Ten, Graft-versus-Host Disease, for more about your eyes and chronic GVHD.)

Bone Loss

Loss of bone density (osteoporosis) sometimes occurs after transplant. It is most common in people who are:

- female
- older
- post-menopausal
- inactive
- have a small frame
- treated with steroids

If your bone density is low, your doctor may recommend:

- exercise
- calcium
- vitamin D

- hormone replacement therapy
- bisphosphonate

Avascular necrosis (joint deterioration) occurs in five-to-ten percent of transplant survivors, particularly those exposed to prolonged high dosages of steroids. It usually affects the hips, but can occur in the shoulder and ankles as well. Surgery is often used to correct the problem.

Many transplant centers now routinely measure calcium and vitamin D levels in the first year after transplant and adjust supplements as needed.

Kidneys

Kidney disease can occur following transplant. The risk of kidney disease is greatest among patients who were treated with total body irradiation.

Treatment for kidney disease varies depending on the particular type of kidney problem you have. If you have kidney problems, be sure to talk with your doctor about all medications you take, including herbal supplements, as some can make the problem worse.

Lungs

Bronchiolitis obliterans is a disease that can develop in the lungs as a result of chronic graft-versus-host disease. Approximately one-in-six patients with chronic GVHD develops this problem.

Bronchiolitis obliterans makes it difficult to breathe and, if left untreated, can be life-threatening. Since symptoms of bronchiolitis obliterans often do not occur until the disease has progressed, frequent pulmonary function tests after transplant are important to help you catch this problem before it becomes severe.

Some chemotherapies, such as bleomycin and carmustine, as well as radiation, can cause scarring in the lungs. Surgeries to remove infections and radiation may affect breathing as well.

Think of exercise as a vital sign and report any changes in exercise tolerance to your doctor. Your doctor may order tests to determine changes in lung function.

Avoid smoking, including e-cigarettes and marijuana, and limit your exposure to vapors in the work place.

Liver

Iron overload is a problem for 25-50 percent of transplant recipients. Iron overload is caused by multiple red blood cell transfusions that deposit excess iron in the tissues.

Your doctor can check your ferritin level and other blood tests to determine if you have excess iron in your body. An MRI may be needed to look for iron overload because other medical problems can cause an increased level of ferritin as well. Medications are available to help your body get rid of iron or your doctor may recommend removing some blood from you periodically (phlebotomy).

Neuropathy

Neuropathy is a nerve condition that sometimes occurs after transplant. Neuropathy can cause pain, numbness or tingling in the hands and feet. The discomfort may be greater at night or in cold weather.

Some drugs used during or after transplant can cause peripheral neuropathy. These include:

- cisplatin
- vincristine
- thalidomide
- lenalidomide (Revlimid®)
- bortezomib (Velcade®)
- brentuximab vedotin (Adcetris®)

Even if you did not receive one of these drugs, you may have neuropathy from your combination of treatments.

(Watch a video about managing neuropathy at bmtinfonet.org/video/managing-neuropathy-after-transplant.)

Dental Problems

Twice-a-year dental cleaning and oral exams are an important part of your long-term health care. After transplant, a dentist or doctor should examine your mouth, including your tongue, for any signs of tissue changes that could be cancer.

Decreased saliva production may occur after transplant and can increase the risk of tooth decay and gum disease. Chronic graft-versus-host disease can cause dental problems as well and increases the risk of mouth cancer.

Prescription toothpastes with high flouride content, such as Prevident®, or fluoride rinses provided by your dentist may aid in preventing these complications.

Frequent follow-up with a dentist is important to prevent serious dental issues.

(For more on management of dental problems caused by chronic graft-versus-host disease go to Chapter Ten, Graft-versus-Host Disease.)

Fertility and Sexual Health

Most, but not all, transplant survivors will be infertile after transplant, especially those who received busulfan (Myleran® or Busulfex®) or total body irradiation as part of the preparative regimen. The risk of infertility is less with reduced intensity or nonmyeloablative transplants. (For more on infertility and options for creating a family after transplant see Chapter Eighteen, Family Planning.)

Sexual difficulties are common after transplant, but are often not discussed by patients and physicians. Physical as well as psychological factors can contribute to problems with intimacy after your transplant.

Since treatment for sexual changes are most effective when they are addressed early after transplant, ask for help as soon as you notice that you are having difficulty. (See Chapter Seventeen, Sexual Health after Transplant for a more detailed discussion.)

Secondary Cancers

Transplant survivors have an increased risk of developing a new cancer. The risk increases over time, so it is important to have regular cancer screening tests as part of your annual exams.

- Breast cancer sometimes occurs in patients who had radiation therapy to their chest.

- Patients who had chronic GVHD, as well as some who did not, have a higher risk of developing skin, mouth and thyroid cancer than the general population.

Screening guidelines for transplant survivors are similar to those recommended for the general population. However, women who received radiation to the chest should have a mammogram at age 25 or eight years after transplant, whichever comes later, and before age 40.

All transplant survivors should guard against exposure to the sun, especially those who had total body irradiation or skin graft-versus-host disease.

- When outside, wear a hat, long sleeves and pants.

- Use a strong sunscreen (SPF30 or higher) on any exposed skin.

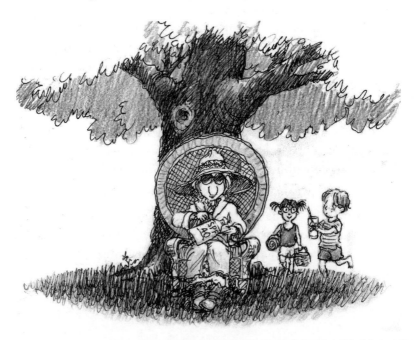

- Keep in mind that the sun's rays can be just as damaging on a cool, cloudy day as they are on a hot, sunny day.

Companies like Sun Precautions® and Coolibar® offer sun protective clothing that can help shield your skin from the sun's harmful ultraviolet rays. The makers of RIT Dye make SunGuard™, a laundry detergent additive that will add sun block to your everyday clothing.

Relapse

Sometimes a patient's disease comes back after transplant. This is called relapse. Your risk of relapse depends on factors such as:

- the type and stage of your disease prior to transplant
- the number of years since transplant

If you relapse after transplant, your doctor can advise you on available treatment options. A second transplant may be an option or you may be eligible for a clinical trial testing new drugs or therapies.

Thoroughly examine your options so you can make a choice that is right for you. Don't be afraid to get a second opinion. Different institutions may have different treatment options or clinical trials to offer you.

Late Effects in Children

Growth Problems

Some children experience slow or stunted growth after transplant. The problem occurs most often in children who received total body irradiation prior to transplant.

If your child was age ten or less at the time of transplant, growth hormone replacement therapy may help spur growth. Growth hormone therapy does not typically improve height in children who were older than ten at the time of transplant.

A thyroid hormone deficiency can also affect your child's growth and may not show up until two or more years after transplant. Your child should be tested regularly to ensure that this is not an issue.

Learning and Organizational Challenges

Many children who have had a transplant do well in school after transplant. However, some children experience learning difficulties after transplant and will need special accommodations at school.

Learning problems are more common among children transplanted at an early age and those who had total body irradiation. Problems may include:

- difficulty remembering things
- poor eye-hand coordination
- problem solving difficulties
- difficulty sustaining attention
- organizational problems

A pediatric neuropsychologist can test your child for learning disabilities and help you obtain any necessary accommodations your child may need at school to succeed academically. Similar tests help teens and young adults identify professions that match their learning and performance skills.

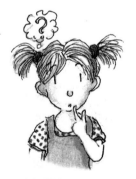
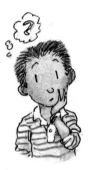

Puberty and Fertility

Most girls who are transplanted during or after puberty experience ovarian failure or premature menopause and will be infertile, due to high-dose chemotherapy or radiation.

If your child retains her fertility after transplant, she may have a higher than normal risk of problems during pregnancy including:

- premature delivery

- cesarean section delivery
- an infant with a low birth weight

However, infants born to women who had a transplant as a child are as healthy as those born to women who did not undergo a transplant.

Boys who are transplanted before puberty typically maintain normal testosterone levels. However most boys, regardless of age, will be infertile, due to high-dose chemotherapy or radiation.

If your child retains his fertility after transplant, his offspring will not have a higher risk of health problems than the general population.

Dental Problems

Children transplanted before the age of five may experience significant dental problems, such as loose teeth, tooth loss and dry mouth and may be unable to wear braces. It is important that they be followed by a dentist who is experienced in treating children who've undergone high-dose chemotherapy or total body irradiation.

Heart Problems

Some chemotherapy drugs used prior to transplant, such as doxorubicin, daunorubicin and mitoxantrone, can damage a child's heart muscle cells. Total body irradiation can also increase the risk of heart problems later in your child's life.

Although there may be no symptoms of a heart problem for several years, your child may receive an echocardiogram every one to five years to monitor for heart problems.

Take Charge of Your Health

Your transplant has given you a new lease on life. Protecting your health requires a life-long commitment to regular check-ups, reporting new problems to your doctors, and being persistent in getting the care you need to address any health issues.

Lifestyle changes can make a big difference in your long-term quality of life. Regular exercise, a good diet and limiting the stress in your life can help you make the most of your second chance at life.

Learn more about potential late complications after transplant at:

bmtinfonet.org/late-effects

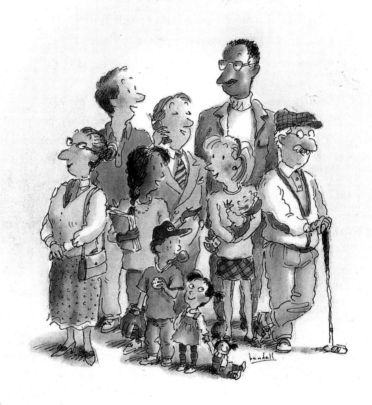

Chapter Seventeen

SEXUAL HEALTH AFTER TRANSPLANT

No one ever mentioned that my sex life might be affected by transplant. It wouldn't have changed my decision to have a transplant, but it sure would have prepared me better for what to expect and what to do about it.

Robert, 12-year transplant survivor

It's the elephant in the room: sexual difficulties after transplant. No one talks about it upfront, especially when life and death matters are of primary concern.

Although pop culture is full of sexy images and dialogue, a frank and honest discussion about sex is not something that is encouraged. Many people feel embarrassed to even bring it up with their doctor, and physicians are equally uncomfortable discussing it with patients. Hence, the topic often goes unaddressed and patients suffer in silence.

But changes in sexual health after transplant are common and knowing what to expect and how to deal with these changes can ease distress between partners.

Not everyone experiences changes in sexuality after transplant. However, in one study by Syrjala et al, 46% percent of men and 80% percent of women reported lower sexual activity and sexual function five years after transplant than those who had not had a transplant. Women who resumed sexual relations during the first year after transplant appeared to have less difficulty later than those who did not.

Changes in sexuality may come as a surprise for both you and partner alike. Fortunately, if sexual difficulties do arise there are several things you can try to do to remedy the situation and make sex a pleasure once again.

Talking openly with your partner about any changes in desire, arousal or sexual satisfaction that you are experiencing is important. You will need to work together to address the problem, and communicating about these issues will help you develop a plan.

The solution may mean changing the way you seek and enjoy intimate relations. A consultation with a trained sex therapist can be helpful in identifying ways to regain intimacy.

What Causes the Change?

Both radiation and chemotherapy can impact sexual function after transplant. Depression, mood changes and some antidepressants and pain medicines can also affect sexual health. Patients who develop graft-versus-host disease on their genitalia may also experience sexual difficulties.

Males

Men who undergo total body irradiation (TBI) may experience damage to the small blood vessels in the penis. This can make it difficult to achieve an erection. Radiation and some types of high-dose chemotherapy can cause nerve damage, and a reduced level of testosterone can decrease desire.

Difficulty achieving an erection can be treated by medications such as Viagra®, Cialis® or Levitra®. These drugs relax smooth muscle cells that let blood flow into the penis. However, they don't work as well if nerves have been damaged, and they do not increase desire.

Injections of drugs such as Caverject® and Edex® can help men achieve erections. Vacuum devices, although cumbersome, are also very helpful.

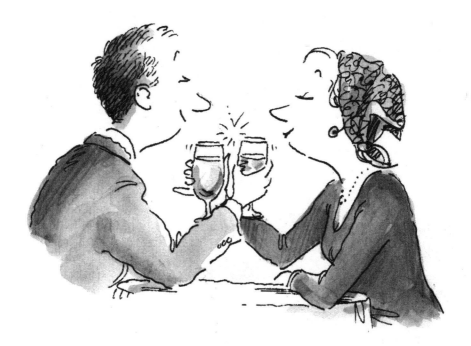

Talk with your doctor about whether these or other therapies, such as surgical implants, are appropriate for you.

Most men recover normal testosterone levels between six months and two years after transplant. For those who continue to have low or low-normal testosterone levels, testosterone replacement can help.

Watch a helpful video about male sexual health after transplant at bmtinfonet.org/video/mens-sexual-health-after-transplant.

Females

Radiation and high-dose chemotherapy usually cause premature ovarian failure. Women who undergo a reduced intensity transplant have a lower risk of premature ovarian failure than those who undergo a standard transplant.

Ovarian failure reduces the ability of the vagina to stretch, and reduces the lubricating fluid in the vagina.

- The vaginal skin becomes thin and fragile.
- During intercourse there can be bleeding, soreness or burning.
- Pain, as well as menopausal symptoms like hot flashes and reduced testosterone, can reduce a woman's desire for intercourse.

Many women report decreased physical arousal, difficulty reaching orgasm or orgasms that are not as intense as they used to be before transplant. Vaginal graft-versus-host disease can cause vaginal scarring which makes intercourse painful or impossible.

There are various therapies that can be used to address these problems:

- Vaginal moisturizers such as Replens®, K Y Liquibeads® or similar products used regularly can be useful.

- Water or silicon-based lubricants specifically designed for use before intercourse can also help.

- Some women find that a vaginal dilator improves blood flow to and elasticity of the vagina

Many women experience early menopause following transplant. Hormone replacement therapy can be useful, although it has been controversial in recent years. A discussion with your doctor about the risks and benefits of this therapy will help you decide whether it is right for you.

Watch a helpful video about female sexual health after transplant at bmtinfonet.org/video/women's-sexual-health-after-transplant.

Psychological Issues

Aside from the physical difficulties created by transplant, psychological issues can also affect your sexual desire and pleasure.

- Both you and your partner may worry about infection, particularly if your immune system has not fully recovered.

- Weight loss or weight gain, scars, temporary hair loss and other physical changes can affect how you feel about your body and sexual appeal.

Some people find that taking it slow and easy helps them transition back into a satisfactory sexual relationship. There are a variety of different techniques one can use to achieve intimacy with a partner. A sex therapist can help you identify some new techniques to try.

> The most important thing is to maintain honest, open communication with your partner about what both of you need and can achieve. Don't assume you know what your partner wants.

Find a time when you are both relaxed but not in the middle of sexual activity to discuss how things have changed. Discuss cues (such as moving a hand) or words to communicate what you like or don't like. This can eliminate frustration and misunderstanding and accelerate the road to sexual recovery.

Resources

The American Society of Sex Educators, Counselors and Therapists can refer you to a certified sex therapist in your area. Find a therapist online at aasect.org or phone 202-449-1099.

Will2Love.com is an online resource designed to help cancer survivors regain sexual health after transplant.

Woman Lab offers videos and information about sex and cancer at womanlab.org/category/sex-and-cancer.

To learn more, go to our website at:

bmtinfonet.org/sexual-health-after-transplant

Chapter Eighteen
FAMILY PLANNING

Deciding to undergo a transplant was the hardest decision of my life. The odds of survival were not in my favor, and the fact that I would be infertile after the transplant tore me apart. I finally decided I had too much to live for, and too much more to accomplish to give up. I agreed to have the transplant.

Lisa, seven-year transplant survivor

Most, but not all, patients who undergo a blood stem cell transplant will be infertile afterward. The likelihood of infertility depends on:

- your age
- gender
- sexual maturity
- type and amount of chemotherapy and/or radiation you receive as part of the preparative regimen

Fortunately, there are options available for couples who wish to have children after transplant.

- Medically-assisted reproduction is one option.
- Adoption is another option.

Understanding the options in advance of your transplant will enable you to better plan for children after transplant, and relieve some of the stress associated with the prospect of infertility.

Medically-Assisted Reproduction

Couples who wish to bear children after transplant may benefit from recent advances in medically-assisted reproduction technology. While not always successful, assisted reproduction allows women who are infertile to bear children, and men to contribute to the genetic make-up of their child.

Artificial Insemination

Artificial insemination is a procedure in which male sperm are injected into a woman's vagina at the point in her monthly cycle when a mature egg is most likely to have been released into the fallopian tube. If the sperm fertilizes an egg and the resulting embryo implants in the lining of the uterus, a pregnancy begins.

Frozen sperm have been successfully used in artificial insemination. Thus, if you are facing the possibility of infertility post-transplant you may wish to bank some of your sperm prior to transplant.

If your sperm is not frozen prior to transplant, it is still possible for you and your partner to have a child using donor sperm. A donor may be someone you know or sperm from a sperm bank.

In-Vitro Fertilization

Women who are infertile after transplant may be able to carry a child to term with the help of in-vitro fertilization (IVF). IVF enables eggs to be fertilized by male sperm in a laboratory dish. The resulting embryos are then transferred to the woman's uterus. If an embryo implants in the uterine lining a pregnancy begins.

IVF can be done using your own eggs that were collected before transplant or eggs donated by a friend, relative or anonymous donor. Although in-vitro fertilization with donated eggs does not allow you to contribute to the genetic make-up of your child, you can carry and nurture the child in your womb during pregnancy, and mother it thereafter.

For men who have a very low sperm count or low sperm motility after transplant, intracytoplasmic sperm injection (ICSI) is a potential treatment option. In this procedure, a reproductive specialist

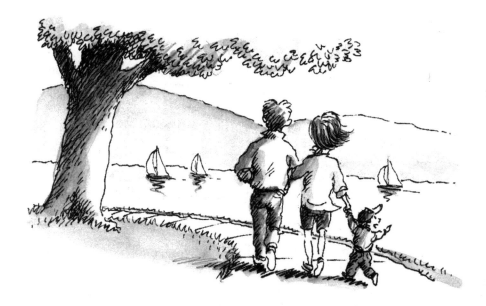

inserts a single sperm into the egg to fertilize it. The egg is then implanted in the woman's uterus.

In-vitro fertilization is expensive and insurance may or may not cover the cost. It can take several cycles before in-vitro fertilization is successful, and for some couples, it may not be successful at all. Nonetheless, many transplant survivors have succeeded in becoming pregnant after transplant with the help of in-vitro fertilization.

To learn more about assisted reproduction techniques, contact:

Livestrong® Fertility
855-220-777
livestrong.org/we-can-help/fertility-services

American Society for Reproductive Medicine
205-978-5000
reproductivefacts.org

The Oncofertility Consortium
866-708-3378
oncofertility.northwestern.edu

Adoption

People who have been treated for a life-threatening illness may find it difficult to adopt a child in the U.S. through a traditional adoption agency. Most adoption agencies have strict requirements regarding the health history of adopting parents and may deny you because of your prior illness or treatment.

However, it may be possible to arrange for a private domestic adoption. Hiring a skilled adoption attorney to help you is recommended. An adoption attorney can:

- prevent you from making costly mistakes
- advise you what is allowed under state law
- help you to publicize your interest in adopting a child

Contact the American Academy of Adoption & Assisted Reproduction Attorneys at 317-407-8422 or visit their website adoptionart.org to find a reputable adoption attorney.

Adopting a child from a country other than U.S. is another option to consider. Each country has its own guidelines regarding the adoptive parents' health history, which may be less restrictive than those of domestic adoption agencies.

Many transplant survivors have successfully adopted children after transplant and are enjoying their role as parent to the fullest.

To learn more, go to our website at:

bmtinfonet.org/build-family-after-transplant

Appendix A

ABOUT BLOOD CELLS

Blood is composed of many different kinds of cells, each with a specific function. Most blood cells are formed in the bone marrow and released into the bloodstream at various stages of maturity. In healthy adults, an estimated 500 million new blood cells are produced each hour.

During your treatment, the medical team will be monitoring the level of various types of blood cells. Those that you will hear about most often are red blood cells, white blood cells and platelets.

Red blood cells (erythrocytes) pick up oxygen in the lungs and transport it to tissues throughout the body. They also pick up carbon dioxide from tissues, and transport it back to the lungs where it is exhaled.

White blood cells (leukocytes) are needed to fight infection. The main types of white blood cells and their functions are described on the next page.

Platelets (thrombocytes) are the smallest cell elements in the bloodstream. Platelets are needed to control bleeding.

All blood cells evolve from primitive cells in the marrow called pluripotent stem cells. Pluripotent stem cells are unique cells that can replicate themselves as well as produce two other types of stem cells called myeloid stem cells and lymphoid stem cells. These stem cells, in turn, either replicate themselves or produce other cells that eventually evolve into blood cells.

A group of white blood cells called lymphocytes evolve from lymphoid stem cells. Red blood cells, platelets and other types of white blood cells evolve from the myeloid stem cell.

White Blood Cells

There are five main types of white blood cells: lymphocytes, monocytes, neutrophils, eosinophils and basophils.

Lymphocytes are the smallest white blood cells. Lymphocytes fight viral infections and help destroy bacteria, fungi and other parasites.

One type of lymphocyte — the T-cell — is the body's main defense against viruses and protozoa.

A second type — the B-cell — produces proteins called antibodies. The antibodies attach to the surface of foreign organisms or the cells they've invaded. They then summon another group of proteins, called "complement" to surround the organism or infected cell and dissolve a hole in it.

Monocytes are the largest white blood cells. They can surround and destroy invading bacteria and fungi. They also clean up the debris that is left after other white blood cells destroy foreign organisms.

When monocytes leave the bloodstream and enter tissues or organs, they can evolve into larger cells called **macrophages**. Macrophages have an even greater ability to destroy foreign organisms that invade the body.

Neutrophils (also called granulocytes) fight bacterial infections. They patrol the body via the blood stream or lymph system, seeking out and destroying harmful bacteria. (The lymph system is a network of vessels that run alongside the blood stream.)

Eosinophils attack protozoa that cause infection.

Basophils are the least common type of white blood cell and their function is not completely understood. They play an important role in regulating allergic reactions such as asthma, hives, hay fever and reactions to drugs.

Blast Cells

White blood cells pass through several stages of development before maturing into lymphocytes, monocytes, neutrophils, eosinophils or basophils. Very immature white blood cells are called blast cells or blasts.

Blast cells are usually found only in the bone marrow. If a large number of blast cells are detected in the bloodstream, you most likely have leukemia. A smaller number of blasts are sometimes detected in the bloodstream of patients who are recovering from chemotherapy or an infection. This is common and is not an indication that you have leukemia.

Appendix B

UNDERSTANDING BLOOD TESTS

Have you ever wondered what all those blood tests were measuring? Here's a guide to help you make sense of the results.

Complete Blood Count (CBC)

Describes the number, type and form of each blood cell. It includes all tests described below.

Red Blood Cell Count (RBC)

Counts the number of red blood cells in a single drop (a microliter) of blood. Normal ranges vary according to age and sex.

Men: 4.5 to 6.2 million
Women: 4.2 to 5.4 million
Children: 4.6 to 4.8 million

A low RBC count may indicate anemia, excess body fluid or hemorrhaging. A high RBC count may indicate polycythemia (an excessive number of red blood cells in the blood) or dehydration.

Total Hemoglobin Concentration

Hemoglobin gives red blood cells their color and carries oxygen from the lungs to cells. This test measures the grams of hemoglobin in a deciliter (100 ml) of blood, which can help physicians determine the severity of anemia or polycythemia.

Normal values are:

Men:	14 to 18 g/dl
Women:	12 to 16 g/dl
Children:	11 to 13 g/dl

A significant anemia occurs when the hemoglobin drops below 10 g/dl.

Hematocrit

Hematocrit measures the percentage of red blood cells in the sample. Normal values vary greatly:

Men:	45% to 57%
Women:	37% to 47%
Children:	36% to 40%

Erythrocyte (RBC) Indices

Three indices that measure the size of red blood cells and amount of hemoglobin contained in each.

Mean Corpuscular Volume (MCV) measures the volume of red blood cells. Normal is 84 to 99 f l.

Mean Corpuscular Hemoglobin (MCH) measures the amount of hemoglobin in an average cell. Normal is 26 to 32 pg.

Mean Corpuscular Hemoglobin Concentration (MCHC) measures the concentration of hemoglobin in red blood cells. Normal is 30% to 36%.

White Blood Cell Count (WBC)

Measures the number of white blood cells in a drop (microliter) of blood. Normal values range from 4,100 to 10,900 but can be altered greatly by factors such as exercise, stress and disease.

A low WBC may indicate viral infection or toxic reaction. A high WBC count may indicate infection, leukemia, or tissue damage. An increased risk of infection occurs once the WBC drops below 1,000/microliter, and especially below 500/microliter.

WBC Differential

Determines the percentage of each type of white blood cell in the sample. Multiplying the percentage by the total count of white blood cells indicates the actual number of each type of white blood cell in the sample.

Normal values are:

Type	Percentage	Number
Neutrophil	50-60%	3,000-7,000
Eosinophils	1-4%	50-400
Basophils	0.5-2%	25-100
Lymphocytes	20-40%	1,000-4,000
Monocytes	2-9%	100-600

A serious infection can develop once the total neutrophil count (percentage of neutrophils times total WBC) drops below 500/microliter.

Platelet Count

Measures the number of platelets in a drop (microliter) of blood. Platelet counts increase during strenuous activity and in certain conditions called myeloproliferative disorders. Infections, inflammation, malignancies and removal of the spleen can also cause platelet counts to increase.

Platelet counts decrease just before menstruation. Normal values range from 150,000 to 400,000 per microliter. A count below 50,000 can result in spontaneous bleeding; below 10,000, patients are at risk of severe, life-threatening bleeding.

GLOSSARY OF TERMS

Acute: Having severe symptoms and a short course.

Adjuvant therapy: Additional drug or other treatment designed to enhance the effectiveness of the primary treatment.

ALL: Acute lymphoblastic leukemia.

Allograft: Bone marrow, stem cells or cord blood stem cells from a donor, used in an allogeneic transplant.

Alopecia: Loss of hair.

AML: Acute myeloid leukemia or acute myelogenous leukemia.

Anaphylactic shock: A life-threatening allergic reaction characterized by a swelling of body tissues including the throat, difficulty in breathing, and a sudden fall in blood pressure.

ANC: Absolute neutrophil count.

Anemia: Too few red blood cells in the bloodstream, resulting in insufficient oxygen to tissues and organs.

Anorexia: Loss of appetite.

Antibiotic: A drug used to fight bacterial infections.

Antibody: A protein produced by the body, in response to the presence of a foreign substance, that fights the invading organism.

Antiemetic: A drug used to control nausea and vomiting.

Antigen: A substance that evokes a response from the body's immune system resulting in the production of antibodies or other defensive action by white blood cells.

APL: Acute promyelocytic leukemia.

Ascites: Accumulation of fluid in the stomach area.

Autograft: Bone marrow or stem cells removed from you to be used in an autologous transplant.

Biopsy: Removal of tissue for examination under a microscope, sometimes required to enable the doctor to make a proper diagnosis.

Blast crisis: In patients with chronic myelogenous leukemia, the progression of the disease to an advanced phase, evidenced by an increased number of immature white blood cells in the circulating blood.

BM: Bone marrow.

BMT: Bone marrow transplant.

Catheter: Small, flexible plastic tube inserted into a portion of the body to administer or remove fluids.

CBSC: Cord blood stem cell.

Central line: Central venous catheter.

Central venous catheter: Small, flexible plastic tube inserted into the large vein above the heart, through which drugs and blood products can be given, and blood samples withdrawn.

Chemo: Chemotherapy.

Chemo-responsive: Responds to chemotherapy.

Chromosomes: Physical structures in the cell's nucleus that house the genes. Each human cell has 23 pairs of chromosomes.

CLL: Chronic lymphocytic leukemia.

CML: Chronic myeloid leukemia or chronic myelogenous leukemia.

CMMOL: Chronic myelomonocytic leukemia.

CNS: Central nervous system.

Contracture: Shortening of muscle, skin and other soft tissue, usually in the limbs.

CR: Complete remission.

Cryopreservation: To preserve by freezing at very low temperatures.

CSF: Colony stimulating factor.

CT scan: Also called a CAT scan or CT-X-ray. A three-dimensional x-ray.

Cytokines: Powerful chemical substances secreted by cells. They play an important role in regulating the immune system.

DFS: Disease free survival.

ECG: Electrocardiogram.

Edema: Abnormal accumulation of fluid. For example, pulmonary edema refers to a build-up of fluid in the lungs.

EFS: Event-free survival.

EKG: Electrocardiogram.

Electrocardiogram: Test to determine the pattern of a patient's heartbeat.

Electrolyte: Minerals found in the blood such as potassium that must be maintained within a certain range to prevent organ malfunction.

Foley catheter: Flexible plastic tube inserted into the bladder to provide continuous urinary drainage.

Glucose: A sugar found in blood.

Hb: Hemoglobin.

HBV: Hepatitis B virus.

HCT: Hematopoietic cell transplantation.

HCV: Hepatitis C virus.

HD: Hodgkin disease.

Hematopoietic cells: Cells from which all blood cells derive.

Hemoglobin: The part of red blood cells that carries oxygen to tissues.

Hemorrhage: Bleeding.

HHV6: Human herpes virus 6.

HLA: Human leukocyte antigen.

Hyperpigmentation: Darkening of the skin.

Hypertension: High blood pressure.

Intravenous: In a vein.

IV: Intravenous.

Lipids: Fats.

Low-microbial diet: Special diet designed to reduce a patient's exposure to bacteria.

Lymph nodes: Small bean-shaped organs of the immune system, distributed widely throughout the body.

Lymph: A transparent, slightly yellow fluid that carries lymphocytes, bathes the body tissues, and drains into the lymphatic vessels.

Lymphatic vessels: A body-wide network of channels, similar to the blood vessels, which transport lymph to the immune organs and into the bloodstream.

Malabsorption: Failure of intestines to properly absorb oral medications or nutrients from food.

MDS: Myelodysplastic syndrome.

Metastatic: Spread of a disease from the organ or tissue of origin to another part of the body.

MM: Multiple myeloma.

MRD: Minimal residual disease.

MRI: Magnetic resonance imaging. A method of taking pictures of body tissue using magnetic fields and radio waves.

Myeloablative: Suppresses the immune system

NHL: Non-Hodgkins lymphoma.

NPO: Do not take anything by mouth.

Packed red blood cells: Whole blood minus the plasma.

Palliative: Provides relief rather than a cure.

Pancytopenia: A deficiency of all types of blood cells.

PBSC: Peripheral blood stem cells.

Petechiae: Small red spots on the skin that usually indicate a low platelet count.

Ph: Philadelphia chromosome.

Phlebitis: Inflammation of a vein.

PLT: Platelet.

PR: Partial remission.

Prognosis: The predicted or likely outcome.

Prophylactic: Preventive measure or medication.

QOL: Quality of life.

Relapse: Recurrence of the disease following treatment.

Relapse-free survival: Survival after treatment without relapse.

Remission, complete: Condition in which no cancerous cells can be detected by a microscope, and the patient appears to be disease-free.

Remission, cytogenetic: In persons who had a chromosomal abnormality, a remission with normal chromosomes.

Remission, partial: Generally means that by all methods used to measure the existence of a tumor, there has been at least a 50 percent regression of the disease following treatment.

Renal: Pertaining to the kidney.

RFS: Relapse-free survival.

RSV: Respiratory syncytial virus.

Sepsis: The presence of organisms in the blood.

Serum: The clear liquid that separates from the blood when it is allowed to clot.

Stomatitis: Inflammation of the mouth, tongue or gums.

Subcutaneous: Under the skin.

TBI: Total body irradiation.

Toxins: Agents produced by plants and bacteria normally very damaging to human cells.

Tumor burden: The size of the tumor or number of abnormal cells in the organ or tissue.

Tumor: Uncontrolled growth of abnormal cells in an organ or tissue.

Ultrasound: A technique for taking a picture of internal organs or other structures using sound waves.

Whole blood: Blood that has not been separated into its various components.

Xerostomia: Dryness of the mouth caused by malfunctioning salivary glands.

INDEX

Abdominal pain, 97

Acyclovir, 115, 117

Adcetris® (see Brentuximab vedotin)

Adenovirus, 119

Adoption, 202, 204

Adrenal insufficiency, 180, 182

Adriamycin, 179

Alkeran® (see Melphalan)

Allogeneic transplant, 1, 2-5

Alopecia (see Hair, loss)

American Academy of Adoption & Assisted Reproduction Attorneys, 203

American Association of Sex Educators Counselors and Therapists, 199

American Society for Reproductive Medicine, 203

American Society for Transplantation and Cellular Therapy (ASTCT), 28

Anemia, 182, 209, 210, 214

Antibiotics, 12, 113, 114, 132, 140, 214

Antibody, 111, 121, 206

Antidepressants, 196

Antiemetic, 88

Antithymocyte globulin (ATG), 96, 98

Anthracyclines, 94, 168, 179, 180
Appetite lack of, 97, 102, 131
Arrhythmia, 92
Artificial insemination, 201, 202
Aspergillus, 114-115
ASTCT, (see American Society for Transplant and Cellular Therapy)
ATG (see Antithymocyte globulin)
Ativan®, 140
Atovaqone, 115
Autologous serum tears, 104
Autologous stem cell transplant, ii, 2
Avascular necrosis, 187
Azithromycin, 105

B-cell, 206
Bacterial infection (see Infection, bacterial)
Bactrim® (see Trimethoprim/sulfamethoxazole)
Bandage contact lens, 104
Basophils, 206, 211
Be The Match®
    donor registry, 3, 4, 10, 33
    telephone counseling, 109
    transplant center data, 27
BiCNU® (see Carmustine)
Bilirubin, 91
Bisphosphonate, 187
Bladder
    infection, 113
    irritation, 90
Blast cells (see Blood cells, blast cells)
Bleomycin, 187

Blood and Marrow Transplant Information Network (BMT InfoNet)
    Caring Connections Peer Support Program, ix, 42, 67, 109, 157, 173
    Facebook groups, 173
    long-term follow-up guidelines, 28, 170, 176
    publications, 241-242
    transplant center directory, 20, 25, 27
    website, viii
Blood cells
    blast cells, 207
    counts, 13
    red blood cells (erythrocytes), 8, 91, 205, 206, 209, 210
    white blood cells (leukocytes), 7, 95, 98, 111, 112, 205-207, 210-211
    platelets, 8, 12, 135, 205, 206, 211
    transfusion, 12
Blood pressure, high, 112, 179-180, 218
BMT InfoNet (see Blood and Marrow Transplant Information Network)
Bone loss (see osteoporosis)
Bone marrow
    aspirate, 23, 58, 76, 140
    cells in, 8, 9, 207
    harvest (collection for transplant), 37-38
    definition, 7-8
    transplant, 2-3, 9
Bone marrow harvest (see Bone marrow, harvest)
Bortezomib (Velcade®), 188
BostonSight®, 104
Botanicals to avoid, 134-135
Breathing problems (see Lungs, breathing problems)
Brentuximab vedotin (Adcetris®), 188
Bronchiolitis obliterans, 187
Bronchodilators, 105

Broviac catheter (see Central venous line)
Budesonide, 102
Busulfan (Myleran® or Busulfex®), 86, 90, 189
Busulfex® (see Busulfan)

Candida, 114
Cardiomyopathy, 178-180
Caregivers, 151-166
    caring for physical and mental health. 153-155, 184
    changing relationships, 162-163
    counseling, 109
    emotional health, 153, 155-158, 160, 165-166, 172
    financial challenges, 27
    helping children cope, 164
    required for transplant, 24, 151
    responsibilities and role of, 78, 152, 158-159, 161, 162, 164
    support for, 24, 157
    taking time to recharge, 153
Caring Connections Program, (see Blood and Marrow Transplant Information Network, Caring Connections)
CaringBridge, 161
Carmustine (BiCNU®), 90, 92, 187
Cataracts (see Eyes, cataracts)
Catheter, 215
    central venous, 11, 86, 215
    Foley (bladder), 90
CBC, 209
CellCept® (see Mycophenolate mofetil)
Center for International Blood and Marrow Transplant Research (CIBMTR), 28, 170
Centers for Disease Control (CDC), 121
Central venous line (see Catheter)

Cevimeline (Evoxac®), 102
Chemotherapy, high-dose (see Preparative Regimen)
Child bearing post-transplant (see Fertility and see Infertility)
Children's Oncology Group, 170
Cholesterol, high, 168, 171, 179-180
CIBMTR, (see Center for International Blood and Marrow Transplant Research)
Cisplatin, 188
Clobetasol gel, 102
CMV (see Cytomegalovirus)
Cognitive behavioral therapy
    for fatigue, 183
    for insomnia, 60, 184-185
Cognitive problems, 92, 169,
    attention and memory problems, 181
    confusion, 13, 9, 92, 108
    learning disabilities, 93, 172, 191-192
Colon
    graft-versus-host disease, 104
    infection 118, 133
Complete Blood Count (CBC), 209
Conditioning regimen (see Preparative regimen)
Confusion (see Cognitive problems)
Conscious sedation, 140
Constipation, 126, 133
Contractures, 101, 102
Cord blood
    access to units, 33
    transplant, 1, 4, 9, 33
Coronavirus, 119
Corticosteroids, 102

side effects, 169, 186, 187
used for, 102, 104, 105, 106
Cresembra®, (see Isavuconazonium sulfate)
Cyclophosphamide (Cytoxan®)
side effects, 90, 92, 179
uses for, 96
Cyclosporine, 96, 100
eye drops, 103
Cytomegalovirus, 34, 118
Cytoxan®, (see Cyclophosphamide)

Dapsone, 115
Daunorubicin, effect on heart, 94, 193
Dental problems, (see Mouth, dental problems)
Depression
causes, 108
effect on relationships, 162-163
impact on health, 126, 130, 138, 182, 184, 196
managing, 59-60, 145
Dexamethasone, 102
DFS, (see Disease-free survival)
Diabetes, 39, 168, 172, 177, 179, 180-181, 184
Diarrhea, 87-88, 97, 104, 132-133
Diet, (see Nutrition)
Diflucan® (see Fluconazole)
Dilaudid® (see Hydromorphone)
Disease-free survival, 26
Donor for transplant
being a, 10, 35-43
bone marrow harvest, 37-38
emotional considerations, 42
factors considered when choosing, 38, 39-40

    finding a donor, 31-34
    haploidentical, 31
    HLA type, 32
    impact on donor health, 38
    related, 10, 31
    stem cell harvest, 36-37
    types of, 3
    unrelated, 10, 33
Doxorubicin (Adriamycin®), 94, 168, 179, 180, 193
Dyclone®, 89

Eating difficulties (see also Nutrition)
    changes in taste, 128
    constipation, 133
    diarrhea, 132-133
    dry mouth, 102, 127
    lack of appetite, 97, 130-131
    mouth sores, 89, 102
    nausea and vomiting, 129-130
    thick saliva, 128-129
    total parenteral nutrition (TPN), 126
EBMT, (see European Group for Blood and Marrow Transplantation)
EBV (see Epstein-Barr virus)
ECP (see Extracorporeal photopheresis)
EFS (see Event-free survival)
Electrolytes, imbalance 92, 182
Emotional health, 15 (see also Depression)
    caregiving and, 155-158
    children, 164
    managing, 51-64, 172-174
    stressful side effects of transplant, 57-59
Engraftment, 12, 85

Eosinophils, 206, 211
Epstein-Barr virus, 119
ERISA, 47
Erythrocyte indices, 210
Erythrocytes (see Blood cells, red blood cells)
Etoposide, 90
Eucerin®, 139
European Group for Blood and Marrow Transplantation (EBMT), 28
Event-free survival, 26
Evoxac® (see Cevimeline)
Exercise
    and appetite, 131
    bone density, 186
    caregivers, 155
    change in tolerance, 187
    constipation, 133
    fatigue management, 182-183
    graft-versus-host disease, 102
    pain management, 139, 145, 147, 148-149, 155
    protect heart, 179
    skin GVHD, 102
Extracorporeal photopheresis, 98, 100, 102, 104, 105
Eyes
    autologous serum tears, 104
    bandage contact lens, 104
    cataracts, 90, 186
    chronic GVHD, 103-104
    dry, 103, 186
    excessive tears, 103
    infection, 117, 118
    irritation, redness, pain, 103
    plugging tear ducts, 103

scarring, 103
scleral contact lens, 104
toxoplasmosis, 119

FACT (see Foundation for Accreditation of Cellular Therapy)
Famciclovir, 117
Family planning, 201-204
Fatigue, chronic, 39, 178, 181-184
Feeding, intravenous, 89, 126
Fertility preservation
    freeze eggs, embryos, or ovarian tissue, 93
    sperm banking, 92-93
Filgrastim (Neupogen®), 36
Finances, costs associated with transplant, 27-28, 40
Fluconazole (Diflucan®), 114
Fluid retention, 90
Fluocinonide, 102
Foley catheter (see Catheter, Foley)
Foundation for Accreditation of Cellular Therapy, 20
Fundraising, 50
Fungal infection (see Infection, fungal)

G-CSF (see filgrastim)
Ganciclovir, 115, 118
Graft rejection, 10
Graft-versus-host disease (GVHD), acute, 95-98
    risk factors, 96
    prevention, 96-97
    symptoms, 97-98
    treatment, 98

Graft-versus-host disease (GVHD), chronic, 99-109, 178
    contractures, 101
    coping with stress, 108-109
    eyes, 103-104, 186
    fingernails and toenails, 101
    gastrointestinal tract, 104
    genitals, 105
    hair, 101
    joints, 101-102
    liver, 104
    lungs, 105, 187
    mouth, 102
    muscles, 107
    nervous system, 106
    rare symptoms, 107
    risk factors, 34, 99
    secondary cancer, 190
    skin, 100-102
    sweat glands, 101
    treatment, 99-100
Granulocytes (see Neutrophils)
Growth factors, 12, 140
GVHD (see Graft-versus-host disease)

Hair
    change in color or texture, 101
    loss, 54, 57, 87, 89, 101
Haploidentical transplant, 5, 10, 31, 33, 218
Harvest
    bone marrow, 37-38
    stem cell, 36-37
    impact on health, 38

HCT (see Hematopoietic stem cell transplant)
Heart problems, 177
    arrhythmia, 92
    cardiomyopathy, 178-180
    coronary artery disease, 178
    heart attack, 180, 181
    in pediatric transplant survivors, 94, 172, 193
    protect against, 179, 180
    tachycardia, 92
Hematocrit, 210
Hematopoietic stem cell transplant
    history, 1
    types, 1-2
Hemoglobin, 209
Hemorrhagic cystitis, 90, 218
Herbs, use during transplant, 124, 134-135
Hepatitis, 40
Herpes simplex virus, 116
Herpes zoster virus, 117-118, 142, 148
Hickman catheter (see Catheter, central venous)
HLA (see Human leukocyte antigen)
Hormone replacement therapy, 186, 198
HPV (see Human papilloma virus)
HSCT (see Hematopoietic stem cell transplant)
HSV (see Herpes simplex virus)
Human leukocyte antigen (HLA), 32
Human papilloma virus, 119
Hydromorphone (Dilaudid®), 138
Hyperalimentation (see Feeding intravenous)
Hyperpigmentation (see Skin, dark spots)
Hypnosis, 139, 141, 143, 145, 147, 148

Ibrutinib (Imbruvica®), 100
ICSI (see Intracytoplasmic sperm injection)
Ifosfamide, 90
Imagery, 145, 147, 148, 149
Imbruvica® (see Ibrutinib)
Infection, 111-122
    adenovirus, 119
    aspergillus, 114-115
    bacterial, 112-114
    candida, 114
    coronavirus, 119
    cytomegalovirus, 34, 40, 116, 118
    Epstein-Barr virus, 119
    fungal, 111, 112, 114-115
    herpes simplex, 116-117
    human papilloma, 119
    influenza, 119, 121
    papovavirus, 119
    parainfluenza, 119
    prevention, 119-121
    protozoa, 119, 206
    respiratory syncytial virus, 119
    rhinovirus, 119
    toxoplasmosis, 119
    vaccination, 121-122, 169, 170-171
    varicella zoster virus, 117
    viral, 115-119
Infertility
    adoption, 204
    after pediatric transplant, 192-193
    American Academy of Adoption and Assisted Reproduction Attorneys, 203

    American Society for Reproductive Medicine, 203
    artificial insemination, 202
    freeze eggs, embryos, or ovarian tissue, 93
    in vitro fertilization, 202-203
    intracytoplasmic sperm injection, 203
    Livestrong Fertility, 203
    risk of, 178, 189, 201
    sperm banking, 92-93, 202
    The Oncofertility Consortium, 204
Influenza virus, 119
Insomnia, 60, 108,178, 182, 184-186
Insurance
    accelerated life insurance benefits, 48-49
    approval for transplant, 45-46
    denial of coverage for transplant, 46-48
Intercourse, painful, (see Sexual health)
Interleukin-2, 100
Intracytoplasmic sperm injection, 203
Intravenous feeding (see Feeding, intravenous)
In vitro fertilization, 201-203
Isavuconazonium sulfate (Cresemba®), 115
IVF (see In vitro fertilization)

Jakafi® (see Ruxolitinib)
Jason Carter Clinical Trials Program, 98
Jaundice, 40, 90, 98, 104
Joints
    deterioration, 187
    stiffness, 101, 102

Kepivance®, (see Palifermin)
Kidneys, 2, 107, 187

    damage, 134
    disease, 187
    excess protein in urine, 107
    fluid retention, 91
    infection, 119
    test, 9, 171

Learning difficulties (see Cognitive Problems)
Lenalidomide (Revlimid®), 188
Leukemia & Lymphoma Society, 83
Leukocytes (see Blood cells, white blood cells)
Lidocaine, 102, 106, 139
Life insurance benefits, 48-50
Liver, 90-91
    damage, 90, 134
    disease, 40, 91
    elevated liver enzymes, 90, 91, 98, 104
    graft-versus-host disease, 98, 104
    jaundice, 40, 90, 98, 104
    infection, 118
    iron overload, 188
    sinusoidal obstruction syndrome, 91
    toxoplasmosis, 119
Livestrong Fertility, 203
Lomotil®, 88, 141
Long-term survivors (see Survival long-term)
Lungs
    breathing problems, 91, 92, 101, 105, 187
    bronchiolitis obliterans, 187
    graft-versus-host disease, 101, 105, 107
    infection, 112, 113, 114, 115, 118, 119
    pulmonary function test, 105, 171, 187

    pneumonia, 92, 112, 114, 115, 118, 119
    scarring, 187
    toxoplasmosis, 119
Lymphocyte (see also White blood cell), 111, 206, 211
Lymphoid stem cell, 205

Macrophages, 206
Marital stress, 65, 77-79, 175
Massage, 22, 102, 106, 139, 145, 148
MCH (see Mean corpuscular hemoglobin)
MCHC (see Mean corpuscular hemoglobin concentration)
MCV (see Mean corpuscular volume)
Mean corpuscular hemoglobin, 210
Mean corpuscular hemoglobin concentration, 210
Mean corpuscular volume, 210
Melphalan (Alkeran®), 179
Memory problem (see Cognitive problems)
Menopause premature, 192, 198
MESNA®, 90
Metabolic problems, 177, 180
Methotrexate, 96, 100
Mini transplant (see Nonmyeloablative transplant)
Mitoxantrone, 94, 193
Monocytes, 206, 207, 211
Morphine, 89, 117, 137, 138, 139
Montelukast. 105
Mouth
    changes in taste, 57, 102, 128
    dental problems, 94, 171, 188-189, 193
    difficulty swallowing, 13, 102, 104, 126-127
    dry, 94, 102, 127, 171, 193
    redness and lacey patches, 102

    sensitivity, 102
    sores, 13, 57, 87, 89, 102, 126-127, 139, 142
    thick saliva, 128-129
Mucositis (see Mouth sores)
Muscle
    contractures, 101
    cramping, 88, 92
    spasms, 92
    weakness, 107, 179
Mycophenolate mofetil (CellCept®), 96, 98, 100
Myeloid stem cell, 205
Myleran® (see Busulfan)

National Marrow Donor Program®, (see also Be The Match®), 10, 33
Nausea, 13, 37, 86, 87-88, 97, 104, 123, 129-130
Nerve damage, 93, 106, 138, 14, 188, 196
Neupogen® (see Filgrastim)
Neuropathy, 93, 106-107, 141, 178, 188-189
Neutropenia, 111
Neutrophils, 111, 206, 211
Nonmyeloablative transplant (see also Reduced intensity transplant), 5, 87, 189
Noxafil® (see Posocanasole)
Numbness in feet and hands (see Neuropathy)
Nutrition, 123-135
    after transplant guidelines, 125
    changing diet before transplant, 124-125
    nutritional needs of transplant patients, 123
    parenteral (see Feeding intravenous)

Opioid, 129, 133, 138, 139, 140, 142, 143
Osteoporosis, 172, 186-187
Ovarian failure, 192, 197

Pain, 137-150
    addiction to medication, 144
    medications to control, 137-144
    non-drug interventions, 145-149
Palifermin (Kepivance®), 89
Papovavirus, 119
Parainfluenza virus, 119
Patient controlled analgesia machine, 143
PCA (see Patient controlled analgesia machine)
Pediatric transplant, 65-83
    behavioral problems, 71
    challenges for parents, 76-77
    concerns of siblings, 68-69, 77
    dental problems after, 94, 193
    growth problems after, 94, 191
    heart problems, 94, 193
    learning and organizational challenges, 93, 191-192
    preparing child for medical procedures, 70, 75
    puberty and fertility, 192-193
    questions children ask, 69-70
    returning home, 79-83
Pentamidine, 115
Peripheral blood stem cell transplant, 1, 5, 9
Pilocarpine (Salagen®), 102
Platelets (see Blood cells, platelets)
Pluripotent, stem cell, 205
Pneumocystis carinii (see Pneumocystis jirovecii)
Pneumocystis jirovecii, 115

Pneumonia, 92
    bacterial, 112
    fungal, 114, 115
    viral, 118, 119
Positive coping statements, 145
Posocanasole (Noxafil®), 115
Prednisolone, 98, 102
Prednisone, 98, 100, 104
Preparative regimen, 11, 85-94
    chemotherapy, high-dose, 11, 86, 13-14
    total body irradiation (TBI), 86-87
    side effects, 13-14, 87-94, 189
PROSE, 104
Protozoa, 119
Psoralen, 98
Psychiatric and psychological counseling, 22, 59, 109, 156, 173, 174, 176
Pulmonary function test (see Lungs, pulmonary function test)

Quality of life after transplant, 176, 193

Radiation (see Total body irradiation)
Rapamune® (see Sirolimus)
Rapamycin (see Sirolimus)
Raynaud's Phenomenon, 107
RBC (see Blood cells, red blood cells)
Red blood cells (see Blood cells, red blood cells)
Red blood cell count (RBC), 209
Reduced intensity transplant, 5, 12, 93, 112, 189, 197
Relapse
    fear of, 62, 172, 174
    risk of, 97, 191
    treatment, 169, 191

Relationships
    marital, 65, 77, 162-163, 175
    friends, 61, 62
Relaxation, 60, 139, 145, 146, 147, 148, 149
Reproductive organs, damage to, 92
Respiratory syncitial virus, 119
Revlimid® (see Lenalidomide)
Rhinovirus, 119
Ribavirin, 119
RSV (see Respiratory syncitial virus)
Ruxolitinib (Jakafi®), 98, 100

Salagen® (see Pilocarpine)
Saliva, thick (see Mouth, thick saliva)
Scleral contact lens, 104
Secondary cancers, 177, 189-190
Sedation, conscious, 140
Sedatives, 76, 87
Septra® (see Trimethoprim/sulfamethoxazole)
Sexual health, 189, 195-199
    achieving erection, 196
    achieving orgasm, 198
    American Society of Sex Educators, Counselors and Therapists, 199
    ovarian failure, 197
    pain during intercourse, 197
    psychological issues, 198-199
    testosterone, low, 197

Shingles (see Varicella zoster virus)
SHINGRIX®, 117
Silvaderm™/Lidocaine®, 139
Sinusoidal obstruction syndrome (SOS), 91-92

Sirolimus (Rapamycin, Rapamune®), 96, 98, 100
Skin
    blisters, 97, 116, 117
    burning sensation, 100, 139, 197
    change in color, 90, 101
    itching, 100, 105, 106, 117, 141
    rash, 90, 97, 100, 117, 141, 142
    sores, 139
    thinning, 101
    tight, taut, 100-101
    yellow, (see Jaundice)
Sleep problems (see Insomnia)
Sleepio.com, 185
Society for Behavioral Sleep Medicine, 185
Sperm banking, 92-93, 201
Stem cells
    collection/harvest, 36-37
    engraftment, 12, 85,
    lymphoid, 205
    myeloid, 205
    pluripotent, 205
    sources of, 9
Steroids (see Corticosteroids)
Stress (see Emotional health)
Survivor guilt, 174
Survivorship care plan, 168-170
Sweat, inability to, 101
Syngeneic transplant, 2

T-cell, 206
    depletion, 97
Tacrolimus, 96, 100, 102, 104, 105, 106

Taste change in (see Eating Problems)
TBI (see Total body irradiation)
TENS (see Transcutaneous electrical nerve stimulation)
Thalidomide, 188
Thiotepa, 90
Throat sores, 89, 126-127, 128
Thrombocytes, 205
Thyroid problems, 177, 180, 182, 191
Toenails, 90, 101
Total body irradiation, 86-87
Total hemoglobin concentration, 209
Total parenteral nutrition (see Feeding intravenous)
Toxoplasmosis, 119
TPN (see Total parenteral nutrition)
Transcutaneous electrical nerve stimulation, 141
Transplant centers,
    accreditation, 20
    choosing, 19-29
    directory of, 20, 25
    success rates, 25-26
Transplant, long-term follow-up
    guidelines, 28
    late effects, 177-194
Triage Cancer, 48, 184
Triglycerides, high, 189-180
Trimethoprim/sulfamethoxazole (Bactrim®, Septra®), 115

Umbilical cord blood transplant (see Cord blood, transplant)
Ursodeoxycholic acid, 104

Vaccination after transplant, 121-122, 171
Vaginal dryness, itching, scarring, 105

Valcyclovir (Valtrex®), 117
Varicella zoster virus (VZV, shingles), 111, 117, 148
Velcade® (see Bortezomib)
Veno-occlusive disease, (see Sinusoidal obstruction syndrome)
Versed®, 140
Vfend® (see Voriconazole)
Viatical settlement, 48-50
Vincristine, 188
Viral Infection (see Infection, viral)
Viruses, 115-119
Vitamin D, 186, 187
Vitamin E, 92
VOD (see sinusoidal obstruction syndrome)
Vomiting, 87-88, 97, 104, 129-130
Voriconazole (VFend®), 114
VZV (see Varicella zoster virus)

WBC (see White blood cell count)
WBC differential, 211
Weight gain, 198
Weight loss, 104, 124, 130-131, 198
White blood cell, 205-207
White blood cell count, 210
Will2Love, 199
Woman Lab, 199
Work after transplant, 15, 59

Zostavax®, 118

Did You Know There is More Useful Literature Published by BMT InfoNet?

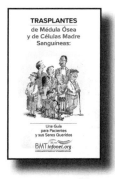

This book, **Bone Marrow and Stem Cell Transplants: A Guide for Patients and Their Love Ones** is also available in Spanish.

Graft-versus-Host Disease: What to Know, What to Do

This free booklet explains the types, symptoms and treatments for graft-versus-host disease. Available in English and Spanish.

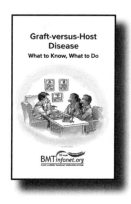

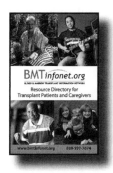

Resource Directory: Tired of searching the web for organizations that can help? Our free **Resource Directory for Patients** does the work for you! We've assembled information about nearly 100 organizations that provide information about transplantation, specific diseases and/or financial aid for transplant patients.

Call us at 888-597-7674 or visit our website at: bmtinfonet.org/products for more details.

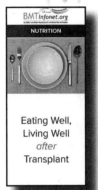

Eating Well, Living Well after Transplant: This brochure offers tips on how to manage eating difficulties that are common after transplant. Available in English and Spanish.

Helpful Hints for Caregivers: This pamphlet provides practical tips for managing the emotional and physical challenges of caring for a transplant patient. Available in English and Spanish.

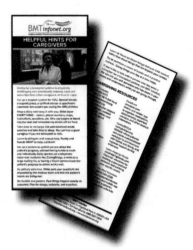

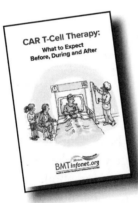

CAR-T Cell Therapy:
What to Expect Before, During, and After
This brochures explains the new immuno-therapy called CAR T-cell therapy. Learn who is a candidate for CAR T-cell therapy, what's involved and whom it helps.

Visit us online at bmtinfonet.org
Email us at help@bmtinfonet.org or call
888-597-7674.